MCQs for ENT:

Specialist Revision Guide for the FRCS

D1354934

MCQs for ENT:
Specialist Revision Guide
for the FRCS

STUART WINTER

DECLAN COSTELLO

ROGAN CORBRIDGE

OXFORD
UNIVERSITY PRESS

OXFORD
UNIVERSITY PRESS

Great Clarendon Street, Oxford OX2 6DP

Oxford University Press is a department of the University of Oxford.
It furthers the University's objective of excellence in research, scholarship,
and education by publishing worldwide in

Oxford New York

Auckland Cape Town Dar es Salaam Hong Kong Karachi
Kuala Lumpur Madrid Melbourne Mexico City Nairobi
New Delhi Shanghai Taipei Toronto

With offices in

Argentina Austria Brazil Chile Czech Republic France Greece
Guatemala Hungary Italy Japan Poland Portugal Singapore
South Korea Switzerland Thailand Turkey Ukraine Vietnam

Oxford is a registered trade mark of Oxford University Press
in the UK and in certain other countries

Published in the United States
by Oxford University Press Inc., New York

British Library Cataloguing in Publication Data
Data available

Library of Congress Cataloguing in Publication Data
Data available

Typeset by Cepha Imaging Private Ltd., Bangalore, India
Printed in Great Britain
on acid-free paper by
Clays Ltd, Bungay, Suffolk

ISBN 978–0–19–953394–7

10 9 8 7 6 5 4 3 2 1

CONTENTS

MCQs for ENT:
Specialist Revision Guide for the FRCS

This book is intended as a revision aid for candidates preparing for the MCQ papers of the FRCS (ORL-HNS) examination. The style and format of the questions in the book mirrors the format of the examination questions, and covers all of the relevant topics.

The book is divided into two main sections: Single Best Answers (SBAs) and Extended Matching Items (EMIs). The SBA section is further divided into chapters by topic: basic sciences; general otolaryngology; rhinology and facial plastic surgery; otology and neuro-otology; head and neck; and paediatric ENT.

Answers and explanatory notes are provided, along with links to relevant websites and key journal articles. In common with the examination, the book features illustrations and diagrams.

1   **Stimulation of which of the following nerves does NOT cause referred otalgia?**

A   Glossopharyngeal nerve
B   Descendens hypoglossi nerve
C   Vagus nerve
D   Lingual nerve
E   Buccal nerve

2   **Parasympathetic innervation to the submandibular gland is carried by the:**

A   Lesser petrosal nerve
B   Facial nerve
C   Glossopharyngeal nerve
D   Jacobsen's nerve
E   Greater superficial petrosal nerve

3   **Which of the following statements BEST describes the physiological regulation of saliva?**

A   Basal saliva production is predominantly from the parotid gland.
B   Parasympathetic stimulation decreases salivary flow.
C   The parotid gland contains largely mucinous cells.
D   Saliva is produced in two stages and its ionic content modified by the intercalated duct cells.
E   Anti-cholinergic drugs increase the production of saliva.

4   Which of the following statements BEST describes the physiology of olfaction?

A   The primary neuron cell body for the 1st cranial nerve is located in the olfactory bulb.

B   Noxious stimuli from the posterior nasal cavity are detected by the glossopharyngeal nerve.

C   The vomeronasal organ detects tactile sensation from passing odorants.

D   Each olfactory receptor expresses only one G protein receptor.

E   Olfactory receptor neurons do not regenerate.

5   What is the single MOST common cause of an incorrect blood transfusion being administered?

A   Laboratory error

B   Error in blood donor centre

C   Minor antigen reaction

D   Clerical error by doctor

E   Failure in pre-transfusion bedside checking

6   Concerning the development of the ossicular chain which statement BEST describes the first branchial arch derivatives?

A   The stapes develops from the first branchial arch.

B   The malleus and incus develop from the first branchial arch.

C   The head and neck of the malleus, and the body and short process of the incus develop from the first branchial arch.

D   The manubrium of the malleus and the long process of the incus develop from the first branchial arch.

E   The head of the malleus and the long process of the incus develop from the first branchial arch.

7   Concerning the pharmacokinetics of local anaesthetics, which of the following statements is FALSE?

A   Lidocaine acts to reversibly block sodium channels in the nerve fibre.

B   Lidocaine acts to cause vasoconstriction when injected subcutaneously.

C   Alcoholic cirrhosis can reduce the metabolism of bupivocaine.

D   Local anaesthetics with a low pKa have a faster onset of action.

E   8.4% sodium bicarbonate added to 2% cocaine speeds up the onset of action.

8 **Which nerves pass through the superior orbital fissure?**

A II, III, IV and VI

B III, IV, V-2 and VI

C III, IV, V-1 and VI

D II, IV, V-2 and VI

E III, IV, V-1 and V-2

9 **Which of the following muscles do NOT have an attachment to the mastoid process?**

A Digastric

B Splenius capitus

C Longissimus capitis

D Temporalis

E Anterior auricular

10 **Concerning lasers in ENT, which if any of the following statements is FALSE?**

A The 'E' in the LASER acronym stands for Emission.

B The CO_2 laser emits light in the far infra-red spectrum and has a wave length of 10 600 nm.

C The light generated by a laser is characterized by being monochromatic, collimated and coherent.

D The effects of the argon laser are due to heat generated locally.

E The KTP laser can be used in middle ear surgery and directed into small recesses by bending the laser light with a prism.

11 **Concerning the hyoid bone, which of the following statements is FALSE?**

A The lesser cornu of the hyoid is derived from the second branchial arch.

B The hyoid bone is incompletely ossified at birth.

C The hyoglossus and middle constricter muscles attach to the greater cornu.

D The intermediate tendon of the digastric muscle passes between the bifurcated tendon of the stylohyoid.

E The geniohyoid muscle acts to depress the larynx during swallowing.

12   **Concerning immunoglobulins, which of the following statements is FALSE?**

   A   IgG crosses the placenta.

   B   IgG forms the largest subclass of immunoglobulins.

   C   Immunoglobulins are composed of heavy and light chains.

   D   IgA is secreted into the saliva.

   E   The antibody binding site is found on the heavy chain.

13   **Which of the following statements is TRUE?**

   A   Clostridia are gram-negative anaerobes.

   B   Some species of Clostridia produce an exotoxin that inhibits the sympathetic nervous system.

   C   *Staphylococcus aureus* are gram-positive cocci that are arranged in clusters.

   D   Lancefield Group C Streptococci include streptococcus pyogenes.

   E   *Treponema pallidum* is a gram-positive spirochaete bacterium.

14   **In designing a trial comparing primary surgery against primary chemo-radiotherapy for head and neck cancer, which of the following statements concerning randomization is TRUE?**

   A   The number of patients in each arm will be the same.

   B   The clinician can favour one treatment over another if the patient expresses choice.

   C   The clinician will not be aware of which treatment the patient has received.

   D   The patients in each arm should have similar prognostic factors.

   E   Randomization ensures that there is no bias between the groups.

15   **A new screening test for a squamous cell carcinoma is developed. 150 people were tested in total. Within the whole study 50 patients were known to have the disease. When testing was started 40 patients that tested positive had the disease, while 10 patients that tested positive did not have the disease.**

   Which of the following statements is CORRECT?

   A   The specificity of the test is 80%.

   B   The sensitivity of the test is 80%.

   C   The positive predictive value of the test is 90%.

   D   The negative predictive value of the test is 80%.

   E   The prevalence of squamous cell carcinoma in this study is 40%.

16 **Concerning the p-value, which of the following statements is TRUE?**

A A p-value of 0.001 with a significance level set at 0.05 indicates that the null hypothesis is wrong.

B For a p-value to be significant it must be a value less than 0.05.

C A type I error is to reject the null hypothesis when it is true.

D A p-value of 0.0001 indicates a highly significant clinical finding.

E The null hypothesis should be rejected if the p-value is 0.1 when the significance level has been set at less than 0.05.

17 **Concerning statistical testing which of the following statements is FALSE?**

A Parametric tests make an assumptions about the population distribution.

B Standard error of a population is calculated as the standard deviation divided by the square root of the population size.

C Specificity relates to the number of true positives in a test.

D A type 1 error is to reject the null hypothesis when it is true.

E A type 2 error is to accept the null hypothesis when it is false.

18 **A 73-year-old woman with a history of metastatic hypopharyngeal squamous cell carcinoma presents with lethargy, vomiting, hypotension, and tachycardia. A corrected serum calcium is found to be 3.14 mmol/l (2.12–2.62). Which of the following ECG abnormalities is MOST likely to be found?**

A QRS interval shortening

B QT interval prolongation

C QT interval shortening

D Peaked T waves

E Poor R wave progression

19 **Which of the following statements concerning botulinum toxin is FALSE?**

A It is produced by *clostridium botulinum*, a gram-positive anaerobe.

B Botulinum toxin acts at presynaptic cholinergic neuromuscular end plate by inhibiting the release of acetylcholine.

C Strains of clostridium botulinum produce different antigenic toxins.

D Recovery after administration occurs as the botulinum toxin is degraded by the anticholinesterase enzyme.

E Following repeated administration antibodies may develop that bind to the botulinum toxin inactivating it.

20   Trousseau and Chvostek signs are observed in hypocalcaemia and also…?

A   Hypokalaemia
B   Hyperkalaemia
C   Hypomagnesaemia
D   Hypermagnesaemia
E   Low zinc levels

21   Concerning anti-cancer clinical drug trials which of the following statements is CORRECT?

A   Phase 1 clinical trials usually involve large numbers of patients to test for anti cancer properties.
B   Phase 2 trials will aim to ascertain the response of the cancer to the treatment.
C   A Phase 3 trial testing a new cancer drug will assess its cost-effectiveness.
D   All cancer patients should be included in clinical trials.
E   Patient consent is not required for the inclusion of patients with advanced cancer into phase 1 trials only.

22   Which of the following statements concerning DNA (deoxyribonucleic acid) is FALSE?

A   The base cytosine binds with guanine in DNA.
B   Large parts of the human DNA sequence do not code for proteins.
C   In DNA replication DNA polymerase copies the DNA sequence in a 5' to 3' direction.
D   Each genes DNA sequence codes for one protein.
E   RNA interference is a naturally occurring system that selectively silences individual genes.

23   The optic canal is formed by which bones?

A   Frontal bone
B   Greater wing of the sphenoid
C   Lesser wing of the sphenoid
D   Temporal bone
E   Ethmoid bone

24 **Parathyroid hormone has all of the following effects EXCEPT…?**

   A Increases osteoclastic activity

   B Increases absorption of calcium from the gastro-intestinal tract

   C Increases renal excretion of phosphate

   D Increases renal absorption of calcium

   E Reduces 1,25-hydroxyvitamin D3

25 **In the Gell and Coombs classification, how is allergic rhinitis classified?**

   A Type 1 – immediate

   B Type 2 – antibody-dependent

   C Type 3 – immune complex

   D Type 4 – cell-mediated

   E Type 5 – seasonal

26 **You are asked by the haematologists to perform a local anaesthetic biopsy of a cervical lymph node. The patient, a 45-year-old woman, has had a suspected relapse of her non-Hodgkin's lymphoma. Following her recent treatment, she is known to be thrombcytopaenic. What is the lowest platelet count (in platelets x 10^9/l) that you would consider it acceptable to proceed with the operation?**

   A 10

   B 20

   C 50

   D 100

   E 150

   C 300

27 **Which of the following statements can be considered FALSE with regard to the prion protein and diseases caused by it?**

   A The prion protein is expressed normally in the human brain.

   B Prion diseases can be inherited, occur sporadically, or be infectious.

   C An example of a human prion disease is Gerstmann–Sträussler–Scheinker disease.

   D There is currently no effective treatment for prion diseases.

   E In the UK several thousand deaths have been caused by new variant Creutzfeldt–Jakob disease (nvCJD) in the last decade.

28 A patient with HIV is placed on the waiting list for a
parotidectomy. You are keen to warn the operating
department staff of his infection risk. When the operating list
is printed, which of the following is generally acceptable to use
to highlight his status?

    A HIV positive

    B High-risk

    C AIDS

    D Special

    E None of the above – it is not ethical to highlight his status on a
circulated list.

29 **Which answer BEST describes the content of the cavernous
sinus?**

    A Internal carotid artery, oculomotor, trochlear, abducent and ophthalmic
and maxillary divisions of the trigeminal nerve

    B Internal carotid artery, oculomotor, trochlear, abducent and ophthalmic
and mandibular divisions of the trigeminal nerve

    C Internal carotid artery, superior ophthalmic vein, optic, abducent and
ophthalmic and maxillary divisions of the trigeminal nerve

    D Common carotid artery, oculomotor, trochlear, abducent and ophthalmic
and maxillary divisions of the trigeminal nerve

    E Superior ophthalmic vein, oculomotor, trochlear, abducent and
ophthalmic and maxillary divisions of the trigeminal nerve

30 **In the UK, under the current Department of Health rules,
when a patient is referred with suspected cancer, what is
the maximum number of days (from the date of referral
by the GP) that a patient may wait for their definitive
treatment?**

    A 14 days

    B 28 days

    C 31 days

    D 42 days

    E 62 days

31 **Which of the following is NOT a recognized side-effect of carbimazole?**

A Agranulocytosis
B Derangement of liver function tests
C Alteration in sense of smell
D Rash
E Gastrointestinal symptoms

32 **The junior doctor on your team receives a complaint alleging that he was rude to a patient's daughter. What is the CORRECT course of action?**

A The doctor should write a polite letter of apology.
B You, as the doctor's senior and supervisor, should write an apology on his behalf.
C Pass the letter to the lead clinician in your department.
D Pass the letter to the hospital's complaints department.
E Ask the nursing staff for a written statement about your conduct.

33 **Which of the following elements of blood clotting are inhibited by the administration of warfarin?**

A Factors II, VII, IX, X
B Factors IIa, IXa, Xa and XIa
C Platelet aggregation
D von Willebrand factor
E Factors II, VIII, X

34 **If a mother and a father are both carriers of an autosomal recessive gene, which of the following statements is TRUE?**

A All of their children will have the disease.
B Half of their children will have the disease.
C One quarter of the children will have the disease.
D All the males will have the disease.
E None of the children will have the disease.

35 **A 44-year-old man presents with a depressed left nasal bone following an alleged assault. He is noted to have reduced sensation to the nasal tip. Which nerve is likely to have been affected?**

A   External nasal branch of the anterior ethmoidal nerve

B   Supratrochlear branch of the ophthalmic nerve

C   Infratrochlear branch of the ophthalmic nerve

D   Superior labial branch of the facial nerve

E   Infraorbital nerve

36 **Which intrinsic laryngeal muscle is responsible for vocal cord opening?**

A   Cricothyroid muscle

B   Posterior cricoarytenoid muscle

C   Lateral cricoarytenoid muscle

D   Thyroarytenoid muscle

E   Thyrohyoid muscle

37 **A patient is taking warfarin for paroxysmal atrial fibrillation (PAF). Under what circumstances would it be reasonable to stop the warfarin and administer fresh frozen plasma (FFP) (or factor concentrate) and Vitamin K?**

A   Epistaxis controlled with anterior nasal packing

B   Epistaxis controlled only with posterior and anterior nasal packing

C   Elective admission for endoscopic sinus surgery

D   Pharyngoscopy for globus pharyngeus symptoms

E   Excision of a lipoma

38 **A randomized controlled trial is conducted to evaluate a novel therapy. What level of evidence does this represent?**

A   1a

B   1b

C   2a

D   2b

E   3

1. B.　　The descendens hypoglossi nerve (C1) is a motor nerve. It joins the descendens cervicalis to form the ansa cervicalis, which supplies the strap muscles.

The glossopharyngeal nerve receives sensation from the posterior one-third of the tongue, the tonsils, the pharynx, and the middle ear.

The vagus nerve supplies sensation to the pinna, tympanic membrane, larynx, hypopharynx, valleculae, and the subglottis.

The lingual nerve, a branch of the mandibular division of the trigeminal nerve, supplies sensation from the anterior two-thirds of the tongue. It also carries 'hitch-hiking' taste and parasympathetic fibres from the chorda tympani.

The buccal nerve is also a branch of the mandibular division of the trigeminal nerve, and transmits sensory information from the skin over the buccal membrane and from the second and third molar teeth.

2. B.　　The parasympathetic supply of the submandibular gland is carried by the facial nerve. The chorda tympani branch of the facial nerve exits the skull base via the petrotympanic fissure to enter the infratemporal fossa. It then hitchhikes on the lingual nerve (branch of Vc) to supply taste to the anterior 2/3 of the tongue and provide parasympathetic fibres to the submandibular gland.

The lesser petrosal nerve (continuation of Jacobsen's nerve) is a branch of the glossopharyngeal nerve. It supplies parasympathetic fibres to the parotid gland.

The greater superficial petrosal nerve branches off the facial nerve at the geniculate ganglion and is then joined by the deep petrosal nerve (sympathetic fibres). It passes forward in the pterygoid canal (Vidian canal) to give parasympathetic innervation to the lacrimal, nasal, palatine, and pharyngeal glands.

3. D. Saliva is produced in two stages. Initially it is isotonic, however the ductal cells modify the ionic composition such that the saliva that is secreted has a similar composition to intracellular fluid.

The basal saliva production is predominantly form the submandibular gland (60–70%) with lesser contributions from the parotid (20–30%) and sublingual glands (5–10%).

When stimulated the parotid contributes the majority of saliva production and this is predominantly regulated by parasympathetic stimulation. Therefore anti-cholinergic drugs reduce saliva production.

The parotid gland largely contains serous cells while the submandibular and sublingual glands contain serous and mucinous cells.

4. D. Each olfactory receptor cell expresses only one type of olfactory receptor. However, a given olfactory receptor can bind to a variety of odour molecules with varying affinities.

The primary neuron cell body for the 1st cranial nerve is located in the nasal mucosa. The cell is bipolar, with a dendrite extending to the nasal mucosa. The cell projects unmyelinated axons from the olfactory receptor cells toward the ipsilateral olfactory bulb to make contact with the second-order neurons.

The trigeminal nerve innervates the posterior nasal cavity to detect noxious stimuli.

The vomeronasal organ is a specialized structure located in the base of the anterior nasal septum. It is believed to detect have a role in detecting pheromones.

Olfactory receptor neurons are replaced approximately every 40 days.

5. E. Contrary to popular opinion, it is clinical ward mistakes that account for most erroneous blood transfusions.

6. C. The first arch derivates of the ossicular chain are the malleus (head and neck) and the incus (body and short process). The stapes superstructure, manubrium of malleus and long process of the incus are derived from the second branchial arch.

7. B. Lidocaine acts to cause vasodilatation in common with other local anaesthetics except cocaine, which is a vasoconstrictor.

Local anaesthetics block sodium channels preventing depolarization and the propagation of action potentials.

Amindes, including bupivacaine, are principally metabolized in the liver, therefore cirrhosis can affect its metabolism.

The speed of onset of the local anaesthetic is proportional to the concentration of non-ionized molecules. The lower the pKa, the higher the concentration of non-ionized molecules at a given pH and therefore faster onset of action. Sodium bicarbonate raises the pH and the speed of action.

8. C. The following structures pass through the superior orbital fissure the lacrimal nerve (V-1), frontal nerve (V-1), trochlear nerve (IV), superior ophthalmic vein, nasocillary nerve (V-1), inferior ophthalmic vein, abducent nerve (VI), oculomotor nerve superior division (III), and oculomotor nerve inferior division (III).

9. D. The muscles attached to the mastoid process are the digastric (posterior belly), sternocleoidmastoid, splenius capitus, longissimus capitis, and the anterior, superior, and posterior auricular muscles.

The temporalis is not attached to the mastoid process.

10. E. LASER is an acronym standing for Light Amplification by the Stimulated Emission of Radiation. The light generated is characterized by being all the same colour (monochromatic), parallel (collimated) and in phase (coherent). The effects of all lasers are due to locally generated heat. The KTP laser does have a role in middle ear surgery but is delivered via total internal reflection along an optical fibre and not bent by a prism. The wavelength of the CO_2 laser is 10 600 nm.

11. E. It is the infrahyoid muscles which act to depress the larynx during swallowing.

The hyoid develops from the second and third brachial arches. The lesser cornu form the second arch and the greater cornu form the third.

Ossification begins in the body and greater cornus and is complete in adolescence.

The hyoglossus and middle constricter attach to the greater cornu.

The digastric muscle does pass through the tendon of the stylohyoid.

12. E. The antibody binding site is part of the light chain. IgG is the only immunoglobulin to cross the placenta and makes up the largest subclass of immunoglobulins. These are composed of heavy and light chains. IgA is present in the secretions of the respiratory tract, lacrimal, and salivary glands.

13. C. Clostridia are gram-positive anaerobes. *Clostridium botulinum* produces an exotoxin that inhibits acetylcholine release from parasympathetic muscle nerve endings. *Streptococcus pyogenes* is classified as Lancefield Group A. Group C contains no significant organisms. *Treponema pallidum* is a gram-negative spirochaete bacterium that causes syphilis.

14. D. The main purpose of randomization is that each group will have similar prognostic factors. Randomization would need to be restricted to ensure equal numbers in each group. The clinician cannot exert bias over the selection group. Comparing surgery with chemo-radiotherapy, it will be obvious following treatment which arm the patient was randomized too unless the data is analysed by a blinded researcher. Randomization does not ensure that there is no bias between groups.

15. B. The following table needs to be constructed to answer this question (bold figures are those given in the text).

		SQUAMOUS CELL CARCINOMA		
		Positive	Negative	TOTAL
SCREENING	Positive	**40**	**10**	50
TEST	Negative	10	90	100
	TOTAL	**50**	100	**150**

The specificity of the test is calculated as the number of true negative results divided by the total number of patients without the disease; 90/100 (90%).

The sensitivity of the test is calculated as the number of true positive results divided by the total number of patients with the disease; 40/50 (80%).

The positive predictive value of the test is calculated as the number of true positive results divided by the total number of positive tests; 40/50 (80%).

The negative predictive value of the test is calculated as the number of true negative results divided by the total number of negative tests; 90/100 (90%).

Prevalence is calculated as the number with the disease over the sample size; 50/150 (33%).

16. C. A type 1 error is to reject the null hypothesis when it is true; this often occurs due to a small sample size.

A p-value less than the significant level set indicates that in the test the null hypothesis should be rejected. This is not the same as saying the null hypothesis is wrong. The p-value can be set at any level between 0 and 1 and is only arbitrarily set as less than 0.05 in most studies.

The null hypothesis is rejected if the p-value is smaller than or equal to the significance level.

17. C. Sensitivity refers to true positive test results and specificity to true negative results. Parametric tests make an assumption about the population distribution and assume a Gaussian or normal distribution. The standard error of a population is calculated as the standard deviation divided by the square root of the population size. A type 1 error is to reject the null hypothesis when it is true and a type 2 error is not rejecting the null hypothesis when it is false.

18. C. Hypercalcaemia can result in a variety of symptoms including fatigue, depression, confusion, anorexia, nausea, vomiting, constipation, pancreatitis, and calculi. This can be remembered using the mnemonic 'bones, stones, moans, and psychic groans'. ECG abnormalities include a shortened QT interval.

19. D. Recovery occurs through proximal axonal sprouting and muscle reinnervation by formation of new neuromuscular junction. Botulinum toxin is produced by *Clostridium botulinum*, a gram-positive anaerobic bacterium. Botulinum toxin is broken into seven neurotoxins. The toxin acts by binding to pre-synaptic sites on the cholinergic nerve terminals. This decreases the release of acetylcholine, causing a neuromuscular blockade. The botulinum neurotoxin can be immunogenic and antibodies may develop that can inactivate it.

20. C. Magnesium is the fourth most common cation in the body. The clinical effects of hypomagnesaemia are neuromuscular irritability, CNS hyperexcitability, and cardiac arrhythmias, including Trousseau and Chvostek signs.

21. B. A Phase 1 trial is the first stage in testing a new treatment. The trials are conducted to assess the safe dose range, side effects and effects on the cancer. Phase 1 trials usually include only a small number of study volunteers.

Phase 2 trials are usually larger than phase 1 trials. If a phase 2 trial can show that the new treatment is as good or better than an existing treatment then a phase 3 trial can be started. A phase 3 study is a formal comparison between the treatment results with the new therapy compared with a standard treatment. This may include a comparison of survival or side effects

Clinical trials are certainly important, but it is the patient's choice whether they wish to be included in a trial, and consent is always required.

22. D. The concept that each gene is translated by one messenger RNA into a single protein is now understood to be false. There are in fact many proteins produced from each gene sequence.

The four bases found in DNA are adenine (A), cytosine (C), guanine (G), and thymine (T). Each type of base on one strand forms a complementary base pairing with a base on the other strand. A binding to T, and C binding to G.

The human DNA sequence contains large regions of non-coding base pairs. Only about 1.5% of the human genome consists of protein-coding exons, with over 50% of human DNA consisting of non-coding repetitive sequences. The exact role of these sequences is unknown but may be involved in the regulation of gene expression.

When a cell divides it must replicate the DNA in its genome. The two strands are separated and the enzyme DNA polymerase creates the complementary DNA sequence. This occurs in a 5′ to 3′ direction. Transcription of the genetic sequence into mRNA (messenger RNA) and subsequently into a protein is performed by the enzyme RNA polymerase.

RNAi is an RNA-dependent gene silencing process that is mediated by the RNA-induced silencing complex (RISC). This is a naturally occurring event used to regulate gene expression. The RNA interference pathway has been exploited in experimental biology to study the function of genes. Using this mechanism, researchers can silence the expression of a targeted gene. This has been extremely useful in understanding the physiological role of the gene product. The use of RNAi and silencing of key genes involved in tumour development are being investigated as potential clinical therapeutic options.

23. C. The optic canal is formed by the lesser wing of the sphenoid

24. E. Parathyroid hormone (PTH) acts to increase the circulating levels of calcium. This is achieved by increasing osteoclastic activity, stimulating the kidney to re-absorb calcium and excrete phosphate. It also acts to convert 25-hydroxyvitamin D3 to the active form 1,25-di-hydroxyvitamin D3 which stimulates the absorption of calcium from the gastro-intestinal tract.

25. A. Allergic rhinitis is a type 1 hypersensitivity reaction provoked by re-exposure to a specific type of antigen.

26. C. A normal platelet count is 150–400, but it is generally considered safe to perform surgery at platelet levels of greater than $50 \times 10^9/l$.

27. E. Deaths in the UK attributable to nvCJD total less than 200 at present.

The human prion gene encodes a protein of amino acids and is found in most tissues of the body but is expressed at highest levels in the CNS.

Prion diseases are unique in that they can be inherited, they can occur sporadically, or they can be infectious. They can affect both animals and humans. Examples include Creutzfeldt–Jakob disease (CJD) and Gerstmann–Sträussler–Scheinker (GSS) in humans, bovine spongiform encephalopathy (BSE) in cattle, and scrapie in sheep.

All prion diseases are fatal, with no effective form of treatment currently.

28. B. The theatre staff should be alerted to his high-risk status, but it is not acceptable to state the exact reason.

29. A.

30. E. Maximum cancer waits from time of GP referral:
- 14 days until first appointment with specialist
- 31 days from decision to treat until first definitive treatment
- 62 days until first definitive treatment.

31. B. Relatively common side effects of carbimazole include allergic-type reactions of fever, rash, urticaria and arthralgia. Agranulocytosis is a much-feared but rare complication of carbimazole and propylthiouracil. It occurs in 0.1–0.5% of patients and occurs suddenly. Routine monitoring of full blood count is therefore of little use.

32. D. Every hospital has a complaints department, and all disputes should be referred to them. It may be necessary to provide a written statement about the incident, but this is best handled by that department.

33. A. Vitamin K, in its reduced form, is a cofactor for the enzymatic reaction in which the glutamic acid residues on the amino terminal end of coagulation factors II, VII, IX and X are converted into gamma-carboxyglutamic acid residues.

Warfarin acts as a competitive inhibitor of the reaction in which oxidized vitamin K is turned into reduced vitamin K.

Hence, warfarin inhibits the vitamin-K dependent factors, namely II, VII, IX and X.

Factors IIa, IXa, Xa, and XIa are inhibited by the heparin-antithrombin complex.

Von Willebrand factor is a plasma glycoprotein that acts as a bridge between platelets and damaged subendothelium at the site of vascular injury.

34. C.   Half of the children will be carriers; one quarter will be homozygous for the gene and hence will have the disease; and one quarter will neither be carriers nor have the disease.

35. A.   Sensation to the dorsum and tip of the nose is supplied by the external nasal branch of the anterior ethmoidal nerve (V2). This emerges from between the nasal bones and the upper lateral cartilages.

36. B.   The posterior criocarytenoid muscle is the only abductor of the vocal cords.

37. B.   In the elective situation, the patient's anticoagulation should be discussed with his/her cardiologist. Epistaxis requiring anterior and posterior packing suggests a heavy bleed, and it would be reasonable under these circumstances to reverse the warfarin. If the bleeding is controlled with conventional anterior packing, cessation of the warfarin will suffice.

38. B.   Levels of evidence for studies evaluating therapy, prevention, aetiology or harm:
- 1a Systematic review (with homogeneity) of RCTs
- 1b Individual RCT (with narrow confidence interval)
- 2a Systematic review (with homogeneity) of cohort studies
- 2b Individual cohort study (including low quality RCT; eg < 80% follow-up)
- 3a Systematic review (with homogeneity) of case-control studies
- 3b Individual case-control study
- 4 Case-series (and poor-quality cohort and case-control studies)
- 5 Expert opinion without explicit critical appraisal, or based on physiology, bench research, or 'first principles'.

1   **Which of the following is NOT an opening into the temporal bone?**

A   Internal auditory canal
B   Vestibular aqueduct
C   Jugular foramen
D   Cochlear aqueduct
E   Subarcuate fossa

2   **Which of the following BEST describes Koerner's septum?**

A   The petrosquamous suture
B   The squamotympanic suture
C   The petrotympanic suture
D   The medial limit of the mastoid antrum
E   The bony covering of the sigmoid sinus

3   **An auditory brainstem implant is being inserted into a patient with neurofibromatosis type 2. Where is the target region for the implant?**

A   On the floor of the third ventricle
B   The cochlear nucleus
C   The Olivary complex
D   The vestibular nuclei
E   The inferior colliculus

4 **When performing a middle cranial fossa approach for an acoustic neuroma, which of the following is the LEAST useful surgical landmark?**

A Middle meningeal artery

B Greater superficial petrosal nerve

C Arcuate eminence

D Bill's bar

E Foramen ovale

5 **Which answer BEST describes the anatomy of the vestibular system?**

A The superior vestibular nerve is anterior to the facial nerve in the internal auditory canal.

B Surgical division of the superior vestibular nerve is a recognized treatment for BPPV.

C Vestibular Evoked Myogenic Potentials (VEMPs) exploit a vestibulocolic reflex whose afferent limb is the superior vestibular nerve.

D The utricle principally senses linear acceleration in a horizontal plane.

E The principle arterial supply to the vestibular organs is from the middle meningeal artery.

6 **Which of the following statements BEST describes electrophysiological brainstem response audiometry?**

A The Auditory Brainstem Response (ABR) is a measure of the cochlear response to a stimulus.

B During Auditory Brainstem Response (ABR) testing wave one (I) represents activity in the cochlear nucleus.

C Electro Cochleography (ECoG) provides an accurate assessment of auditory thresholds at low frequencies.

D Electro Cochleography (ECoG) can accurately test for Ménière's disease.

E Cortical Evoked Response (CER) audiometry requires the non-test ear to be masked.

7 **Cochlear anatomy and physiology. Which of the following statements is FALSE?**

A Endolymph has an electrolyte composition similar to intracellular fluid (high potassium and low sodium ions).

B There are equal numbers outer and inner hair cells.

C The inner hair cells receive 95% of the afferent innervation from the cochlear nerve.

D The sterocillia act as mechanical tranducers.

E Inner hair cells are arranged in a single row.

8 **A man has been sitting on a playground roundabout facing the centre of rotation and travelling in a clockwise direction. When the roundabout stops he has fast beating nystagmus to the right. Which of the following statements is correct?**

A He has ampullopetal flow of endolymph in his left superior semicircular canal.

B He has ampullopetal flow of perilymph in his left posterior semicircular canal.

C He has ampullopetal flow of endolymph in his right horizontal semicircular canal.

D He has ampullofugal flow of perilymph in his right horizontal semicircular canal.

E He has ampullofugal flow of endolymph in his right horizontal semicircular canal.

9 **Which of the following statements BEST describes otoacoustic emissions (OAEs)?**

A OAEs represent sound generated by the outer hair cells.

B OAEs are usually present in children with glue ear.

C A positive test is subjective based on the interpretation of the result.

D In neonatal screening the demonstration of OAEs excludes severe SNHL.

E Evoked OAEs are generated by all normal cochleas.

10 **A 45-year-old man undergoes speech audiometry. Which of the following statements is FALSE?**

A   Speech audiometry frequently uses spondees; that are phonetically balanced words.

B   The Speech Recognition Threshold (SRT) is the quietest level that an individual can repeat half of the spondees.

C   If the patient developed glue ear it is likely that his maximal discrimination score will remain the same.

D   Speech audiometry can always detect feigned hearing loss from true threshold change.

E   'Roll over' of the speech audiogram is associated with retrocochlear pathology.

11 **Concerning noise-induced hearing loss, which of the following statements is MOST appropriate?**

A   The inner hair cells are more susceptible to damage than the outer hair cells.

B   Intermittent noise exposure is more harmful than continuous noise exposure at a similar frequency and intensity.

C   Noise-induced hearing loss occurs because a temporary threshold shift does not occur.

D   Hair cell re-generation takes up to 10 years.

E   A 10 dB increase in sound level involves a 10-fold increase of the sound intensity.

12 **The owner of a Birmingham car factory approaches you. His workers are exposed to a continuous constant level of noise. He wishes to know at what level he needs to provide ear protectors?**

A   75dBA

B   80dBA

C   85dBA

D   90dBA

E   95dBA

13 **Which statement BEST describes the underlying genetic problem in neurofibromatosis 2?**

A It is an inherited autosomal dominant syndrome. There is over-expression of the tumour suppressor gene on chromosome 22.

B It is an inherited autosomal dominant syndrome. There is over-expression of the tumour suppressor gene on chromosome 17.

C It is an inherited autosomal recessive syndrome. There is over-expression of the tumour suppressor gene on chromosome 22.

D It is an inherited autosomal recessive syndrome. There is decreased expression of the tumour suppressor gene on chromosome 22.

E It is an inherited autosomal dominant syndrome. There is decreased expression of the tumour suppressor gene on chromosome 22.

14 **A patient is on your operating list for a right stapedotomy. Which of the following would cause you MOST concern?**

A Suppurative ear discharge

B A tympanic membrane perforation

C Cochlear otosclerosis on the CT scan

D Previous stapes surgery

E A dead left ear

15 **A 46-year-old man presents to the Accident and Emergency department following a head injury with a clear discharge from his right ear. Which of the following statements concerning Beta 2 transferrin and CSF leaks is FALSE?**

A Beta 2 transferrin is unique to the CSF.

B The test requires only a small volume.

C Beta 2 transferrin can be detected even in the presence of contamination with blood.

D Beta 2 transferrin has a high sensitivity and specificity in diagnosing CSF leak.

E The test involves an electrochemical diffusion gradient.

16 In the recovery room following a modified radical mastoidectomy, the patient is found to have a facial nerve palsy. The surgeon was confident that she had not injured the nerve during the operation. What would be the MOST appropriate next action?

A   Immediately re-explore the ear

B   Give steroids in recovery

C   Wait for the local anaesthetic to wear off

D   Ask a colleague to re-explore the ear immediately

E   Arrange a CT scan

17 Which nerve is LEAST likely to be affected in a patient with a lesion involving their jugular foramen?

A   Vagus nerve

B   Cervical sympathic chain

C   Spinal accessory nerve

D   Glossopharyngeal nerve

E   Hypoglossal nerve

18 You are called to the Accident and Emergency department to see a 26-year-old girl who has taken an overdose of aspirin within the last 24 hours. She has developed tinnitus and has hearing thresholds of 50dB bilaterally. Previously she reports normal hearing. What advice would you give her?

A   In the long term her hearing is likely to remain constant with thresholds of 50dB.

B   Her hearing is likely to get worse over the next few months.

C   Early consideration of a cochlear implant will give her the best chance of functional recovery.

D   Her hearing is likely to improve.

E   She is likely to need a bone conduction hearing aid in the long term.

19 A 22-year-old male presents with left pulsatile tinnitus. A CT is arranged. What is the likely diagnosis?

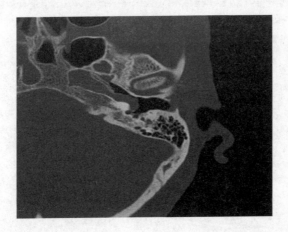

A   Cholesteotoma

B   Glomus tympanicum

C   Glomus jugulare

D   Persistent stapedial artery

E   Carotid body tumour

20 A 46-year-old male has an MRI scan due to asymmetrical sensioneural hearing loss and paresthesia of his left ear canal. A high resolution T2W MRI demonstrates a large left-sided tumour in the cerebellar pontine angle returning mixed signal. What is the likely cause for the altered sensation?

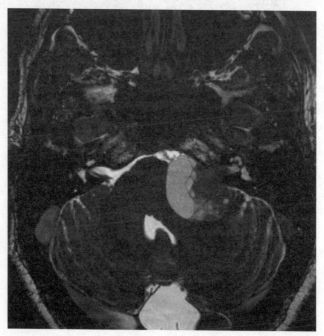

A Compression of the superior vestibular nerve
B Compression of the inferior vestibular nerve
C Compression of the cochlear nerve
D Compression of the facial nerve
E Compression of the vagus nerve

21 What is the MOST common histopathological finding associated with congenital deafness?

A Cochlear aplasia
B Loss of the bony division between the apical and middle turns of the cochlear
C Dysplasia of the membranous labyrinth
D Partial aplasia of the cochlear duct
E Hypoplasia of the stria vascularis

22 **Which of the following statements BEST describes the use of sodium fluoride in the treatment of otosclerosis?**

A The usual dose of sodium fluoride is 1–2g per day.

B Sodium fluoride has no side effects.

C Sodium fluoride is effective at reversing established hearing loss.

D Sodium fluoride is thought to reduce bone resorption.

E Intra-tympanic sodium fluoride administration allows a more accurate dose titration.

23 **The radiological imaging characteristics of a cholesterol granuloma of the temporal bone are BEST described as?**

A Hyperintense on T1 and T2 MRI imaging

B Hyperintense on T1 and hypointense on T2 MRI imaging

C Hypointense on T1 and hyperintense on T2 MRI imaging

D Enhancement following gadolinium-contrast on MRI imaging

E Contrast enhancement on CT scanning

24 **Within the middle cranial fossa the arcuate eminence on the superior aspect of the temporal bone corresponds BEST to which structure?**

A Apical turn of the cochlea

B The epitympanic recess of the middle ear

C The greater superficial petrosal nerve

D The superior semicircular canal

E The lateral aspect of the internal acoustic meatus

25 **A 46-year-old man presents with reduced hearing in his right ear. On examination is he is found to have a single bony mass protruding into the ear canal with a build-up of cerumen and consequent conductive hearing loss. Clinically this is an osteoma. Which of the following statements is the LEAST accurate description for this condition?**

A Osteomas are benign tumours.

B They typically develop along the tympanosquamous or tympanomatsoid suture line.

C Surgical removal is curative.

D Histologically they are described as being composed of mature lamellar bone with bone marrow.

E They are commonly associated with a history of cold water exposure.

26 **Concerning the outer and middle ear sound transformer mechanisms which of the following is statements is FALSE?**

A The pinna aids in the localization of sound.

B An in the ear hearing aid will generally reduce 2 kHz sounds.

C The ratio of the size of the tympanic membrane to the stapes footplate is important in sound amplification.

D The ossicular chain dampens sound transmission to the inner ear.

E The middle ear transformer mechanism normally results in a 25 dB amplification of sound.

27 **Whilst descending on a SCUBA dive, a 30-year-old man experiences a sudden onset of hearing loss and vertigo. Which of the following BEST describes the mechanism of injury to his inner ear?**

A Rupture of the round window on 'Valsalva' equalization of pressure

B Increased middle-ear pressure on descent

C Ossicular discontinuity

D Tympanic membrane rupture

E Rupture of stapedius tendon

28 **A 25-year-old lady presents with a 4-day history of right-sided facial weakness. On examination she is found to have a House–Brackmann Grade IV facial palsy. No underlying cause is found, and a diagnosis of Bell's palsy is made. Regarding her recovery, what would you tell her?**

A There is a greater than 90% chance of a complete recovery.

B There is approximately a 70% chance of a complete recovery.

C There is approximately a 50% chance of a complete recovery.

D There is approximately a 30% chance of a complete recovery.

E There is approximately a 10% chance of a complete recovery.

29 **Gentamicin is known to be ototoxic. On which part(s) of the inner ear does it exert its toxic effects?**

A Stria vascularis

B Hair cells

C Cochlear nerve

D Apical turn of cochlea

E Macula densa

30 **Which of the following statements regarding clival chordoma tumours is TRUE?**

A The tumour arises from a remnant of the first branchial arch.

B They occur exclusively in the head and neck.

C Primary chemotherapy offers the best chance of survival.

D Clival tumours are usually extradural.

E Clival tumours commonly present with hypoglossal nerve palsy.

31 **Aminoglycocides are recognized to have ototoxic properties. Which of the following statements is CORRECT?**

A Aminoglycocides cause a predominantly low frequency hearing loss.

B Aminoglycocide toxicity is usually spontaneously improves over weeks to months.

C Mutations in the 12S mitochondrial rRNA gene are associated with low dose aminoglycocide ototoxicity.

D Gentamicin is more cochlear toxic than vestibulo-toxic.

E The principal area of damage is the stria vascularis.

32 **Concerning barotrauma following flying, which of the following statements is FALSE?**

A The eustachian tube is normally closed.

B Otalgia on ascent is more common than on descent.

C The volume of air in the middle ear cleft is decreases as atmospheric pressure increases.

D Hearing loss and vertigo can occur due to the pressure changes exerted during flying.

E Air pressure at sea level is 760 mmHg.

33 **Which of the following is NOT an indication for placement of a bone-anchored hearing aid (BAHA)?**

A Congenital ossicular malformation

B Complete absence of the external ear (Grade III microtia)

C Unilateral sensorineural hearing loss

D Bilateral sensorineural hearing loss

E Learning difficulties and a conductive hearing loss

34 **Which of the following statements is TRUE of Carhart's effect?**

A It may occur in glue ear.

B It typically occurs at 4kHz.

C It is not improved following stapes surgery.

D It represents a genuine sensorineural hearing loss which is overcome
with stapes surgery.

E It occurs only in otosclerosis.

35 **Which of the following sounds should be used performing a
visual reinforcement audiogram (VRA)?**

A Warble tones

B Pure tones

C White noise

D Complex sound (e.g. music)

E All of the above

1. C. The jugular foramen is bordered laterally by the temporal bone but does not enter it.

The internal auditory canal transmits the facial nerve, the vestibular nerves and the cochlear nerve.

The vestibular aqueduct transmits the endolymphatic duct.

The cochlear aqueduct transmits a prolongation of the dura mater establishing a communication between the perilymphatic space and the subarachnoid space, and transmits a vein from the cochlea to join the internal jugular .

The subarcuate fossa transmits a small vein.

2. A. Koerner's septum is the petrosquamous suture and is the lateralmost limit of the mastoid antrum. In dissection of the temporal bone, therefore, it is opened medial to the mastoid air cells before entering the antrum.

3. B. The cochlear nucleus lies in the brain stem and is responsible for processing sound signals carried from the ear through the vestibulocochlear nerve. Auditory brain stem implants are electrodes placed in the cochlear nucleus.

NICE guidelines. IPG 108 Auditory brain stem implants – guidance: Jan 2005.

4. E. The middle fossa approach involves identifying all structures except the foramen ovale.

5. D.   The utricle and the saccule both sense linear acceleration. The utricle senses motion in the horizontal plane (forward-backward or left-right movement), while the saccule senses motions in the sagittal plane (up-down movement).

The superior vestibular nerve is postero-superior in the internal auditory canal and the facial nerve is antero-superior.

The inferior vestibular nerve (singular nerve) innervates the posterior semicircular canal. Surgical division of this nerve is used in the treatment of BPPV.

The VEMP reflex is a vestibulocolic reflex whose afferent limb arises in the acoustically stimulable neurons of the saccule. The afferent limb is the inferior vestibular never. The efferent limb innervates the ipsilateral sternocleidomastoid muscle.

The main blood supply to the vestibular end organs is from the internal carotid artery via the labyrinthine artery. This usually arises from the anterior cerebellar artery, superior cerebellar artery, or basilar artery. The middle meningeal artery is a branch of the maxillary artery.

6. E.   Masking is required for ABR and CER but not ECoG testing.

The Auditory Brainstem Response (ABR) is a neurologic measure of the brain stem response to an auditory stimulus. ABR testing generates waveform peaks that are labelled I–VII. Wave I represents the action potential generated in the cochlear nerve.

The ECoG is considered to offer poor reliability at low frequencies below 500Hz. The ECoG has three components, the cochlear microphonic, the summating potential (SP) and the action potential (AP). The SP/AP ratio is used in some centres investigating patients with Ménière's disease. However, an altered ratio is not generally considered to provide an accurate diagnosis.

7. B.   There are three times as many outer hair cells than inner hair cells. The majority of the afferent cochlear nerve terminals (95%) synapse on the inner hair cells and transmit sensory signals. Endolymph does have an electrolyte composition similar to intracellular fluid (high potassium and low sodium ions) whereas the composition of the perilymph is similar to that of extracelluar fluid (high sodium and low potassium ions).

The sterocillia act as mechanical tranducers. Bending of the sterocillia towards the tallest row causes an opening of channels and depolarization. The inner hair cells are arranged in a single row while the outer hair cells are arranged in three rows.

8. C. Angular acceleration is detected by the semicircular canals. The ampulated end of each semicircular canal contains the ampullary crest containing hair cells embedded in the cupula.

When the endolymph moves, the hair cells within the cupula are displaced to one side or the other. Movement of endolymph in the horizontal semicircular canals towards the ampulla (ampullopetal) increases the firing rate, while movement of endolymph away from the ampulla (ampullofugal) results in decreased firing. This is in contrast to the superior and posterior semicircular canals, where ampullopetal flow decreases and ampullofugal flow increases the firing rate.

The horizontal semicircular canals are paired such that increased firing in one canal is balanced by decreased firing in the opposite one.

Thus when a person is rotated clockwise the bony labyrinth rotates clockwise while the endolymph remains 'relatively' static due to inertia. This causes the cupula and its hair cells to bend. When the rotation is stopped, the momentum of the now moving endolymph causes it to continue moving. The hair cells are now bent in the opposite direction. Thus in the right ear the endolymphatic flow is ampulopetal and ampulofugal in the left ear. Right fast-beating nystagmus then occurs.

9. A. Otoacoustic emissions represent sound generated by the outer hair cells, typically in response to a sound stimulus. The emissions are frequently absent in conductive hearing loss and are usually absent in severe SNHL although they do not exclude an absent cochlear nerve. The testing is objective and is therefore used in the universal neonatal screening programme. Evoked otoacoustic emissions are generated in the majority (approximately 90%) of a normal population.

10. D. Speech audiometry can be useful in patients with probable feigned hearing loss but it cannot always discriminate between the two.

Spondees are bisyllabic words that emphasise both syllables. The SRT is the softest level (dB) that an individual can repeat at least 50% of the spondees. The maximal discrimination score is the highest percentage of spondees that an individual can repeat at least 50% of the time. In a conductive deafness this is likely to remain unchanged but require a louder stimulus.

Roll over describes the phenomenon whereby the speech discrimination score deteriorates with increasing loudness. This can be associated with retro-cochlear pathology.

11. E. The decibel scale is calculated based on the $10 \log_{10} lx/lo$, where lx is the sound intensity being measured and lo is a reference intensity. Each 10 dB increase represents a 10-fold increase in the intensity of sound ($\log_{10} 10 = 1$).

The outer hair cells are more susceptible than the inner hair cells. Continuous noise is more damaging than intermittent noise of the same frequency and intensity. Theories concerning noise-induced hearing loss include metabolic exhaustion of the hair cells following the temporary threshold shift that occurs in noise exposure. The hair cells do not regenerate.

12. B. The 2005 Control of Noise at Work Regulations sets the lower exposure level at a daily or weekly personal noise exposure of 80 dB (A-weighted) and a peak sound pressure of 135 dB (C-weighted). The upper exposure action values are a daily or weekly personal noise exposure of 85 dB (A-weighted) and a peak sound pressure of 137 dB (C-weighted). At these levels the employer is required to try to reduce exposure to as low a level as is reasonably practicable by establishing and implementing a programme of organizational and technical measures and provide personal hearing protectors.

13. E. NF2 is an inherited autosomal dominant syndrome The manifestations result from mutations in the NF2 gene located on the long arm of chromosome 22. The gene product known as merlin serves as a tumour suppressor. Decreased function or production of this protein results in a predisposition to develop the NF2 phenotypic tumours.

14. A. The presence of active chronic otitis media is considered an absolute contraindication to many while the other responses represent relative contraindications.

15. A. Beta 2 transferrin is not unique to the CSF and is found in perilymph and vitreous humour. The test involves an electrochemical diffusion gradient and requires only a small volume and is not affected by blood contamination. A positive finding of Beta 2 transferrin is highly sensitive and specific for a CSF leak.

16. C. If the surgeon is confident that the nerve was not injured in the operation, it is reasonable to allow any local anaesthetic to wear off. If the palsy persists, the packing could be removed from the ear.

17. E. The contents of the jugular foramen includes the internal jugular vein, inferior petrosal sinus, the posterior meningeal artery, the cervical sympathetic chain, the glossopharyngeal, vagus and spinal accessory cranial nerves. The hypoglossal nerve is not considered part of the jugular foramen.

18. D. Aspirin typically causes a flat hearing loss and is associated with tinnitus. Typically hearing improves over 2–3 days and the tinnitus resolves.

19. D. The stapedial artery is the artery of the second branchial arch. When it persists it is a branch of the internal carotid artery, passing through the arch of the stapes to become the middle meningeal artery. The latter is normally a branch of the external carotid. The absent foramen spinosum is characteristic.

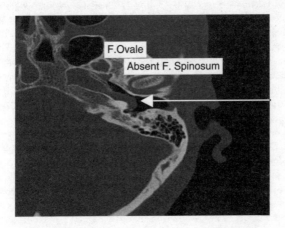

20. D. The axial MRI shows a lesion in the cerebropontine angle. This is likely to be an acoustic neuroma. Altered sensation of the posterior canal skin (Hitzelberger sign) is due to pressure on the sensory fibres of the seventh cranial nerve carried in the nervus intermedius.

21. E. Hypoplasia of the stria vascularis (Scheibe malformation) is the most common histopathological abnormality found in congenital deafness. This abnormality is found in Jervill, Lange–Nielsen, Refsum's, Usher's, and Waardenburg's syndromes.

Cochlear aplasia (Michel malformation is complete failure of development of the inner ear, both membranous and bony aplasia) is a severe abnormality and is rare.

Incomplete formation of the bony and membranous labyrinth, such that the middle and apical turns of cochlea occupy common bony space, is a Mondini malformation. This malformation can be seen in Pendred's syndrome. This may be asymmetrical and auditory function can vary from normal to profound SNHL.

Dysplasia of the membranous labyrinth with a normal bony labyrinth is known as a Bing–Siebenman malformation.

Partial aplasia of the cochlear duct is the Alexander malformation. This results in high frequency hearing loss.

22. D. Fluoride ions replace the usual hydroxyl group in hydroxy apatite. The resulting fluorapatite complex is resistant to osteoclastic bone resorption. The recommended dosage varies but is usually 20–40 mg per day. Side effects include rash, arthritis, and gastrointestinal distress. It is thought that hearing can be stabilized in up to 80% of the population.

23. A. A cholesterol granuloma is characterized having a hyperintense signal character on T1 and T2 MRI imaging and no further enhancement following administration of gadolinium-contrast.

24. D.

25. E. In contrast to exostosis of the external ear canal, osteomas are not generally associated with cold water exposure. They are generally considered to be benign tumours and typically contain mature lamellar bone with bone marrow. Surgical removal is usually curative.

26. D. The pinna has a role in localizing sound. The external ear canal acts as a resonant chamber for sounds in the region of 2 kHz. Therefore 'in the ear' aids dampen sounds at this frequency. The ratio of the tympanic membrane to the stapes footplate coupled with the amplification of sound through the ossicular lever activity results in an amplification of sound.

27. A. On descent, divers should regularly equalise by performing the Valsalva manoeuvre. However, if this is done too forcibly, the sudden change in middle ear pressure can lead to rupture of either the oval or round window.

28. A. Bell's palsy has an almost universally good prognosis: when paralysis is incomplete (as in House–Brackmann Grade IV), function is almost certain to return to normal, whatever intervention is employed.

29. B. Gentamicin is particularly toxic to the first row of outer hair cells in the basal turn of the cochlea. Hence patients experience a high-tone sensorineural hearing loss.

30. D. Chordomas are tumours originating from embryonic remnants of the primitive notochord. The tumour occurs in bone, and so they are usually extradural. They can be found in any part of the axial skeleton but occur most commonly in the sacrococcygeus or clivus. Tumours arising in the clivus cause symptoms due to compression and local invasion. This includes headaches and cranial nerve deficits, the commonest of which is the abducent nerve.

Treatment is surgical were possible with radiotherapy given postoperatively when there is incomplete excision. The tumours are not generally considered to be sensitive to chemotherapy.

31. C. Aminoglycocide ototoxicity is usually causes a high frequency sensorineural hearing loss that is permanent. Damage is usually to the hair cells. Each drug has different affects on the vestibular and cochlear hair cells. Gentamicin is more vestibulo-toxic which has encouraged its use in the treatment of Ménière's. Mutations in the 12S mitochondrial rRNA are associated with low dose aminoglycocide toxicity.

32. B. During ascent middle ear pressure increases and air can passively pass through the eustachian tube. In descent the middle ear pressure reduces and the eustachian tube, which is normally closed, must be actively opened to equalise pressure. A perilymph fistula can occur due to barotrauma and result in hearing loss and vertigo. Boyle's law states that the volume of a gas is inversely proportional to the pressure at a constant temperature.

33. D. A BAHA may be useful in any cause of conductive hearing loss, including complete absence of the external ear. Learning difficulties are not, in themselves, a contraindication to BAHA. Patients with a unilateral, but not bilateral, sensorineural hearing loss may benefit from BAHA.

34. A. Carhart's notch may occur whenever there is a conductive hearing loss. When a bone conductor is applied to the skull, sound reaches the inner ear via the skull and also via the middle ear. This leads to an apparent sensorineural loss when there is a conductive hearing loss. Correction of the middle ear defect results in an apparent improvement in the sensorineural component.

35.A. A visual reinforcement audiogram requires at least 2 testers and a parent to be present. The child sits a table playing with toys and free-field sounds are produced from a loudspeaker on one or other side of the child. If the child responds to the sound by turning towards it, he/she is 'rewarded' by seeing a visual stimulus (e.g. an illuminated toy jumping in a box); this is the 'visual reinforcement'. The child is then presented with sounds of varying intensities and frequencies and hearing thresholds can be ascertained.

See <www.library.nhs.uk/guidelinesfinder/ViewResource.aspx?resID=148627>.

1   In the course of performing a parotidectomy, you are having difficulty identifying the facial nerve. Which of the following would be least useful in identifying the nerve?

   A   Following the posterior belly of digastric
   B   Identifying the tip of the styloid process
   C   Drilling out the mastoid bone
   D   Following peripheral branches proximally
   E   Following the tympanomastoid suture

2   A patient presents with diplopia and nasal obstruction. He is found to have a nasopharyngeal carcinoma that extends though the foramen lacerum into the cavernous sinus. Which of the following is least likely to be affected?

   A   Oculomotor nerve
   B   Trochlear nerve
   C   Ophthalmic division of the trigeminal nerve
   D   Mandibular division of the trigeminal nerve
   E   Sympathetic plexus

3   Your registrar is performing a total laryngectomy without a neck dissection. As part of the dissection he has confidently identified the hypoglossal nerve. He then identifies a further nerve, running in the same direction as the hypoglossal nerve but medial to the common carotid artery. What would you advise him to do next?

   A   Preserve the nerve and continue the dissection.
   B   Dissect the nerve proximally.
   C   Dissect the nerve distally.
   D   Divide the nerve and continue the dissection.
   E   Consider a primary anastamosis after the resection is complete.

4   A 25-year-old professional opera singer attends the voice clinic as an emergency. During last night's performance, she experienced discomfort in her throat and today says that she is struggling to reach high notes. 70° rigid videostroboscopy shows an area of acute haemorrhage on her right vocal cord. What would be the most appropriate advice?

A   Advise her to perform tonight, but sing with less effort.

B   Prescribe prednisolone and advise her to continue with tonight's performance.

C   Advise her not to perform tonight and rest the voice.

D   Advise her to cancel the rest of her 3-month tour.

E   Perform an urgent general anaesthetic laryngoscopy and incise and drain the haematoma.

5   A 60-year-old man presents to the 'lump in the neck clinic' with a 5 cm solitary lymph node in the upper right cervical region and an abnormal-looking right tonsil. Assuming this is a squamous cell carcinoma nodal metastasis, what is the 'N' classification?

A   N1

B   N2a

C   N2b

D   N2c

E   N3

6   A patient presents with a squamous cell carcinoma of the maxillary sinus. Where are the first echelon nodes for this tumour?

A   Intraparotid lymph nodes

B   Preauricular lymph nodes

C   Retropharyngeal lymph nodes

D   Facial nodes

E   Level III lymph nodes

7 **A patient develops a chylous fistula following a left neck dissection. Which of the following treatments is least likely to result in the fistula closing?**

A Endovacular embolization of the thoracic duct

B Enteral diet with containing predominantly medium chain fatty acids

C Surgical re-exploration

D Enteral diet containing predominantly long chain fatty acids.

E Total parenteral nutrition

8 **You see a 46-year-old man with a 3-month history of a mass in the right anterior triangle of his neck. He has smoked 20 cigarettes a day for the last 25 years and drinks in excess of 30 units of alcohol per week. Full ENT examination is otherwise normal. A fine needle aspiration (FNAC) produces 30 ml of milky brown fluid. At 1 week the cyst has re-accumulated and the cytology reports that the fluid contains cholesterol crystals. What is the most appropriate management?**

A Repeat the FNAC.

B Reassure the patient and discharge.

C Commence broad spectrum antibiotics and review in 6 weeks.

D Refer the patient to the oncologists for chemo-radiotherapy.

E Arrange for surgical removal of the cyst along with rigid endoscopy of the upper aerodigestive tract.

9 **Which of the following statements is most appropriate concerning thyroid cancer?**

A Papillary and follicular thyroid carcinomas occur with an equal incidence.

B Follicular thyroid cancers can be diagnosed using fine needle aspiration cytology (FNAC).

C A fine needle aspiration cytology report of a solitary thyroid nodule reported as THY 2 should lead directly on to thyroid surgery.

D Medullary thyroid carcinoma (MTC) associated with the Multiple Endocrine Neoplasia IIb (MEN) carries a better prognosis than that associated with MEN IIa.

E Primary medullary thyroid carcinoma does not occur in a thyroglossal cyst.

10 Following enucleation of a superficial pleomorphic adenoma a patient develops a parotid fistula which discharges onto the cheek. Which is the least effective treatment?

A Repeat aspiration

B Compression

C Vidian neurectomy

D Completion parotidectomy

E Tympanic neurectomy

11 Which of the following statements is true with respect to juvenile nasal angiofibroma?

A It is centred on the sphenopalatine foramen.

B It rarely recurs after excision.

C It occurs predominantly in adolescent females.

D It usually presents with a mass in the neck.

E It has an association with HLA B17.

12 A 45-year-old lady attends the clinic complaining of dry eyes and mouth. You suspect primary Sjogren's syndrome. Which investigation would be most likely to confirm the diagnosis?

A Schirmer's test

B cANCA testing

C ssRho antibody testing

D Rheumatoid factor levels

E Salivary gland biopsy

13 You are called to the Accident and Emergency department to see a 46-year-old male who has been stabbed in the neck with a kitchen knife following a domestic dispute. The knife is still in the neck, entering just above the clavicle on the right side. The patient is haemodynamically stable, talking in complete sentences with no respiratory compromise but is finding swallowing painful. What is the most appropriate next stage of his management?

A Remove the knife and close the wound.

B Remove the knife and explore the wound in the Accident and Emergency department.

C Arrange a contrast radiographic swallow examination.

D Perform an angiogram.

E Perform a barium swallow.

14 A tumour in the pterygopalatine fossa may have developed there primarily or it may have spread directly into the fossa from any of the following except…?

A Orbit through the infra orbital fissure

B The cranial cavity through the foramen ovale

C The cranial cavity through the foramen rotundum

D The nasal cavity

E The oral cavity through the greater palatine canal

15 A 46-year-old man presents with a 5-day history of an upper respiratory tract infection and 2 days' right cervical lymphadenopathy. He is febrile and with a raised white cell count. Ultrasound of his neck reveals thrombus in his right internal jugular vein and a chest x-ray is reported as having changes consistent with 'septic emboli'. Which is the most likely organism responsible for his symptoms?

A *Proteus mirabilis*

B *Clostridium difficile*

C *Fusobacterium necrophorum*

D *Streptococcus pyogenes*

E *Staphylococcus aureus*

16 A carotid body tumour is likely to receive its major blood supply from which vessel?

A Common carotid artery

B Ascending pharyngeal artery

C Superior thyroid artery

D Lingual artery

E Thyrocervical trunk

17 The registrar calls you in for advice. He is performing a rigid
oesophagoscopy on a 38-year-old male with a suspected
food bolus obstruction. He has found a smooth non-pulsatile
indentation on the anterior aspect of the oesophagus at
27 cm measured from the upper incisors. The overlying
mucosa appears normal. What is this likely to represent?

A The cricopharyngeal sphincter

B The left main bronchus

C The aorta

D The gastro-oesophageal junction

E The left atrium

18 A 46-year-old Caucasian male presents with a post nasal space
mass and a 5 cm ipsilateral lymph node. Biopsy of the post
nasal space is reported as non-keratinizing squamous cell
carcinoma. The most appropriate treatment is:

A Radiotherapy to the post nasal space and ipsilateral modified radical
neck dissection

B Chemo-radiotherapy to the post nasal space, ipsilateral modified radical
neck dissection and contralateral selective neck dissection

C Surgical debulking of the post nasal space, bilateral modified radical neck
dissections and post operative radiotherapy

D Primary chemo-radiotherapy

E Palliative care

19 Concerning PET-FDG scanning (positron emission
tomography), which of the following statements is true?

A The radioactive tracer is highly specific for cancer cells.

B PET scanning can define very small tumour deposits of only a few cells.

C PET scanning has an emerging role in the assessment of the unknown
primary.

D PET scanning can differentiate areas of inflammation and cancer deposits.

E PET scanning combined with CT scanning provides improved resolution
of the soft tissues compared to magnetic resonance scanning.

20 **A patient with medullary thyroid carcinoma is also found to have hyperparathyroidism, and genetic analysis reveals a RET proto-oncogene germline mutation. No other physical or biochemical abnormalities are found. What is the most likely diagnosis?**

A Multiple endocrine neoplasia I

B Multiple endocrine neoplasia IIA

C Multiple endocrine neoplasia IIB

D Familial medullary thyroid carcinoma

E Sporadic medullary thyroid carcinoma

21 **As part of completing a modified radical neck dissection you are required to ligate the superior end of the internal jugular vein (IJV). What is the most common relationship to the spinal accessory nerve?**

A The jugular vein commonly splits around the spinal accessory nerve.

B The spinal accessory nerve is medial to the IJV at the skull base.

C The spinal accessory nerve is lateral to the IJV at the skull base.

D The spinal accessory nerve has an equal chance of being medial or lateral to the IJV.

E The spinal accessory nerve is unlikely to be found at the upper end of the IJV.

22 **Concerning obstructive sleep apnoea (OSA), which one of the following statements is true?**

A During sleep muscle tension is maximal during rapid eye movement (REM) sleep.

B The multiple sleep latency test cannot be used to diagnose OSA.

C Pulse oximetry can accurately diagnose OSA.

D The respiratory distress index (RDI) is the number of apnoeas/ hypopnoeas occurring every hour.

E Continuous positive airway pressure (CPAP) is unacceptable first line treatment in a young person.

23   A 24-year-old male **HGV** driver presents with a history of
      snoring, day time sleepiness and obstructive sleep apnoea
      (OSA), confirmed with a polysomnogram. He is hypertensive,
      has a BMI of 30, a neck size of 17 inches and his respiratory
      disturbance index is 18. Which of the following statements
      least accurately describes OSA and its treatment in this
      patient?

A   There may be a direct relationship between his OSA and hypertension.

B   Weight loss is a mainstay of treatment.

C   He should inform the DVLA regarding his condition and cease driving.

D   Uvulopalatopharyngoplasty (UVPP) should be considered as his primary
     treatment.

E   There is good evidence that treating his OSA will improve his quality of
     life and reduce his blood pressure.

24   A 44-year-old female professional singer presents with a
      3-month history of a swelling in her thyroid gland. An initial
      FNA has been reported as Thy 1. A second FNA 6 weeks
      later under ultrasound (US) guidance is reported as Thy 3.
      The US reports a 1 cm nodule in the left thyroid lobe. She is
      biochemically euthyroid and otherwise fit and well. What is
      the next most appropriate management plan?

A   Repeat the FNA.

B   Reassure her and arrange a repeat follow up appointment in 3 months.

C   Arrange for her to undergo a left hemithyroidectomy.

D   Arrange a contract CT scan to exclude a retrosternal goitre.

E   Request serum thyroglobulin levels.

25 **A 47-year-old lady attends your clinic. She is a heavy smoker and is concerned that her voice is low-pitched and occasionally hoarse. Her larynx has the following appearance. You plan to take her to theatre. What is your first priority in her surgical management?**

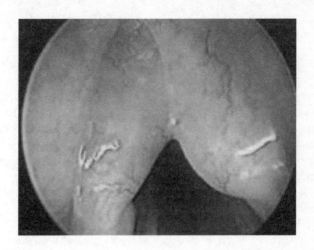

A   Stripping of the vocal cords

B   Incision and drainage of the oedema on one side

C   Incision and drainage of the oedema on both sides

D   Close examination of the post-cricoid region

E   To take biopsies

26 **You are taking consent to proceed with drainage of the oedema in the same 47-year-old lady as in the above question. You explain that you aim to drain the fluid in the vocal cords. Relating to the voice, what affect is this likely to have on her voice?**

A   She may lose her voice altogether.

B   Her voice may go up in pitch.

C   Her voice may go down in pitch.

D   She should not use her voice for 2 weeks post-operatively.

E   Her singing voice will improve.

27 As part of a multidisciplinary team in a voice clinic, which of the following professionals might you **NOT** expect to find present?

A Occupational therapist

B Speech and language therapist

C Manual therapist

D Singing teacher

E Psychologist

28 You are called to see a 44-year-old woman who has undergone a completion thyroidectomy earlier in the day for follicular carcinoma (T2 N0 M0). She is feeling light-headed and short of breath. The FY2 hospital at night doctor has checked her serum biochemistry and performed an ECG, which is normal. She has been prescribed levothyroxine 20µg, tds. There are no other clinical findings. What is the next most appropriate action?

Sodium	137 mmol/l (135–145)
Potassium	4.4 mmol/l (3.5–5.0)
Urea	4.9 mmol/l (2.5–6.7)
Creatinine	89 mmol/l (60–123)
CRP	34 mg/l (0–8)
Bilirubin	8 umol/l (3–17)
ALT	12 IU/l (10–45)
Alk Phos	239 IU/l (110–700)
Albumin	37 g/l (35–50)
Corrected Calcium	2.20 mmol/l (2.12–2.62)

A Start thyroxine (T4) at 100µg/day

B Prescribe calcium gluconate

C Prescribe alpha calcidol

D Reassure her

E Prescribe oral calcium gluconate and re-check the serum biochemistry at 24hours

29 **Which of the following statements best describes the parapharyngeal space?**

A The stylomandibular ligament separates the parapharyngeal space from the submandibular space.

B The foramen ovale opens directly into the parapharyngeal space.

C The parapharyngeal space is divided into pre and post styloid spaces. The pre-styloid space contains the internal carotid artery.

D The majority of primary tumours arising in the parapharyngeal space are benign.

E The pre-styloid space contains the cranial nerves IX–XII.

30 **A laryngeal squamous cell carcinoma has spread from the vocal cord into the pre-epiglottic space. For the tumour to continue to spread anteriorly into the subcutaneous tissues and skin, through which structure will it pass?**

A Epiglottis

B Thyrohyoid ligament

C Thyroepiglottic ligament

D Aryepiglottic fold

E Cricoid cartilage

31 **Concerning the hypopharynx and tumours arising within it, which of the following statements is least likely to be correct?**

A The hypopharynx is defined as extending from the superior aspect of the hyoid to the lower border of the cricoid cartilage.

B Squamous cell carcinomas arising in the post-cricoid region are more common in males.

C Pooling of saliva in the pyriform fossa may be the only sign of pathology using awake flexible endoscopy.

D Tumours arising from the pyriform sinus can spread directly into the paraglottic space.

E A leiomyoma is the commonest benign tumour of the hypopharynx.

32 The following diagram is a schematic representation of the vocal fold. In which layer is a patient most likely to develop Reinke's oedema?

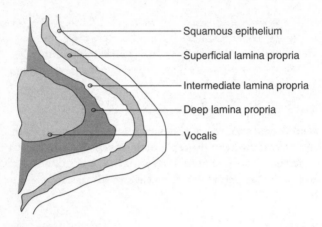

A Squamous epithelium
B Superficial lamina propria
C Intermediate lamina propria
D Deep lamina propria
E Vocalis

33 A 45-year-old female professional vocalist presents with a solitary right thyroid nodule. She is biochemically euthyroid and a full ENT examination is otherwise normal. An FNA is performed and reported as 'Possible follicular neoplasm'. What is the next most appropriate action?

A Reassure the patient and discharge
B Reassure the patient and review in 6 months
C Refer for radioactive iodine
D Screen for a phaeochromocytoma
E Advise right hemithyroidectomy

34 Which of the following is least likely to be improved following orbital decompression for Graves-associated thyroid eye disease?

A Optic neuropathy

B Diplopia

C Exophthalmos

D Cosmesis

E Exposure keratitis

35 A 46-year-old male presents with left-sided nasal obstruction and a single 5 cm left supraclavicular mass. Biopsy of the post nasal space tumour confirms a diagnosis of non-keratinizing nasopharyngeal carcinoma. According to the UICC TNM grading system, what is the correct stage of neck disease?

A N1

B N2

C N2a

D N2b

E N3

36 A 34-year-old man presents with a mass in the right side of his neck in level 5. He is euthyroid, otherwise asymptomatic and a full ENT examination is otherwise normal. A fine needle aspiration is performed and this is reported as 'normal thyroid cells'. What is the most appropriate course of action next?

A Reassure the patient and discharge them

B Reassure the patient and review in 6 months

C Arrange for a lymph node biopsy

D Refer them to the thyroid MDT for a thyroidectomy and neck dissection

E Arrange for radioactive iodine to be administered

37 A 46-year-old, non-smoker patient presents with a long history
    of right-sided throat discomfort. He has no dysphagia and full
    ENT examination is normal. A lateral neck X-ray is requested.

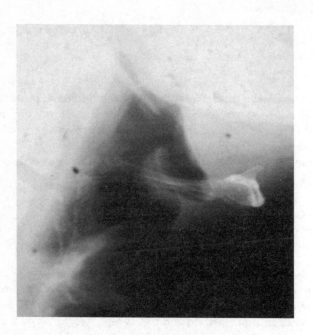

What is the most likely cause for his symptoms?

A Irritation of the vagus nerve

B Irritation of the glossopharyngeal nerve

C Irritation to the hypoglossal nerve

D Irritation to the superior laryngeal nerve

E Irritation to the cervical plexus

38 A 65-year-old woman is found to be hypercalcaemic. In
    locating a parathyroid tumour, which of the following would
    LEAST appropriate imaging modality?

A Ultrasound

B Radio-iodine isotope scanning

C MRI scan of the neck

D Sestamibi scanning

E MRI scan of the chest

39 **Which of the following treatments is least appropriate in the management of medullary thyroid cancer.**

  A Radiation therapy
  B Chemotherapy
  C Radioactive iodine
  D Surgery
  E Prophylactic surgery in childhood

40 **You are taking consent from a 25-year-old lady for excision of a second branchial arch cyst. What risks would it be reasonable NOT to mention?**

  A Paraesthesia to the ear and neck
  B Altered tongue movements
  C Altered facial movements
  D Altered voice
  E Numbness to the cheek

41 **You are counselling a 32-year-old woman about thyroidectomy for her Graves' disease. Which of the following is true?**

  A Her eye symptoms and signs are more likely to improve with radio-iodine than surgery.
  B She would be best served by having a sub-total thyroidectomy.
  C Transient hypocalcaemia is very rare.
  D Superior laryngeal nerve injury is usually asymptomatic.
  E Recurrent laryngeal nerve injury is usually asymptomatic.

42 **A 72-year-old smoker presents to the ENT clinic with a 3-month history of dysphagia and weight loss. Flexible nasendoscopy shows pooling of saliva in the pyriform fossae, with restricted mobility of the right hemi-larynx. Malignancy is suspected. You proceed to general anaesthetic endoscopy. At surgery, you find that he has a 3 cm tumour affecting the right pyriform fossa and extending into the post-cricoid region. According to the TNM staging, what T-stage is this malignancy?**

  A T1
  B T2
  C T2B
  D T3
  E T4

43 A 25-year-old lady presents with a midline neck mass.
Clinically and radiographically, it is a thyroglossal duct cyst.
It is excised in a Sistrunk's procedure, including the middle
one-third of the hyoid bone. Histology shows a papillary
carcinoma in the cyst. Review of the radiology shows no
masses in the thyroid itself or lymphadenopathy. What would
be the most appropriate management of this malignancy?

A External beam radiotherapy

B Subtotal thyroidectomy

C Total thyroidectomy followed by radio-iodine ablation

D Radio-iodine ablation only

E Reassure the patient that the cancer has been excised.

44 A 60-year-old man undergoes a laryngectomy and ipsilateral
neck dissection for a T3 N1 laryngeal carcinoma. Which of
the following would **NOT**, on its own, be an indication for
post-operative radiotherapy?

A Extracapsular spread

B Multiple involved lymph nodes

C Multiple levels of nodes affected

D Maximal lymph node size 3 cm

E Close excision margins

1. B. The tip of the styloid process is variable in position and therefore a poor method for identifying the facial nerve. All of the others are acceptable methods of finding the facial nerve.

2. D. The cavernous sinuses are located at the base of the skull. The internal carotid artery and the sympathetic plexus pass through the sinus. The occulomotor (third), trochlear (fourth), and abducent (sixth) cranial nerves are attached to the lateral wall of the sinus. The ophthalmic and maxillary divisions of the fifth cranial nerve are embedded in the wall. The mandibular division of the of the trigeminal nerve does not pass through the sinus.

3. D. This is likely to represent the superior laryngeal nerve. The superior laryngeal nerve passes along the pharynx medial to the common carotid artery in a similar direction to the hypoglossal nerve. The hypoglossal nerve is lateral to the common carotid artery.

The superior laryngeal nerve separates from the main trunk of the vagus just outside the jugular foramen, it then passes anteromedially on the thyrohyoid membrane where it is joined by the superior thyroid artery and vein. At approximately this level, the external laryngeal nerve leaves the main trunk and the internal laryngeal nerve enters the thyrohyoid membrane.

This nerve is resected as part of performing a laryngectomy.

4. C. She should be advised not to perform tonight and should be reviewed in a few days. It is not necessary to cancel her engagements several months into the future, but she should be closely followed up to ensure resolution of the haematoma.

5. B. Lymph node metastasis from tonsil tumours are classified using the UICC TNM system.
- Nx: Regional lymph nodes cannot be assessed
- N0: No regional lymph node metastasis
- N1: Single ipsilateral lymph node < 3 cm
- N2a: Single ipsilateral lymph node 3–6 cm
  b: Multiple ipsilateral nodes < 6 cm
  c: Bilateral lymph nodes < 6 cm
- N3: Any node > 6 cm

6. C. The nasal cavity first echelon nodes are to the retropharyngeal lymph nodes.

7. D. The majority of ingested fats are triglycerides with long chain fatty acids. Long chain fatty acids are esterified in mucosal cells of the bowel wall and transported into the lymphatic system as chylomicrons.

Middle chain fatty acids, however, are absorbed directly into the portal system without the formation of chylomicrons, bypassing the lymphatics. Therefore dietary modifications avoiding long chain fatty acids are important in the treatment of chylous fistula.

8. E. This is likely to be a branchial cyst. Surgical excision is recommended as the cyst has re-accumulated. Cystic degeneration of a metastatic lymph node remains a possibility, therefore endoscopy of the upper aerodigestive tract should be performed as soon as possible.

9. E. MTC arises from the parafollicular cells (C cells) of the thyroid. Embryologically these are derived from the 5th pharyngeal pouch. The thyroid and hence thyroglossal duct is derived from the 3rd and 4th pharyngeal pouches. Therefore all malignant types of thyroid cancer can arise in the thyroglossal duct except MTC.

80% of thyroid cancers are papillary. Follicular cancer represents 10–15%. FNAC cannot diagnose follicular thyroid cancer.

FNAC are reported as:
- THY 1 – inadequate
- THY 2 – benign appearance
- THY 3 – follicular lesion
- THY 4 – suspicious of malignancy
- THY 5 – malignant cells.

Therefore a THY 2 report may not directly lead on to surgery.

The prognosis of MTC associated with MEN IIb is worse than that associated with all other forms of MTC.

10. C. Vidian neurectomy is performed for the treatment of rhinitis. The vidian nerve carries parasympathetic innervation to the pterygopalatine ganglia and hence to the lacrimal gland and the mucous glands of the nose, nasopharynx and palate.

   The parotid receives parasympathetic innervation from the inferior salivary nucleus. The glossopharyngeal nerve conveys these fibres to the tympanic plexus (Jacobson's nerve) and then lesser petrosal nerve. The postganglionic parasympathetic fibres from the otic ganglion then pass to the parotid gland in the auriculotemporal nerve.

11. A. Juvenile nasal angiofibroma (JNAs) typically arise in the sphenopalatine foramen, which they expand. The occur almost entirely in adolescent males and may recur after resection. Nasopharyngeal carcinoma, when seen with HLA B17, is associated with short-term survival.

12. E. The diagnosis of Sjogren's syndrome can be confirmed by demonstrating peri-ductal fibrosis on biopsy of minor salivary glands. The other tests listed may help to support the diagnosis, but only the biopsy will confirm it.

13. D. For penetrating neck injuries the neck is divided into 3 zones. Zone 1 extends from the clavicle to the cricoid cartilage, zone 2 lies between the cricoid cartilage and the angle of the mandible and zone 3 from the angle of the mandible to the base of skull.

   The injury described is in zone 1. Penetrating neck injuries in this region have a high risk of damage to the carotid and vertebral vascular tree. Furthermore, injuries in this zone can be difficult to control when bleeding occurs with retraction of vessels into the mediastinum. Therefore in a haemodynamically stable patient with a high risk of vascular injury a four vessel angiography is appropriate.

   Other structures that are at risk include nerves traversing the neck including the recurrent laryngeal nerve and the aerodigestive tract. These represent less of an immediate risk to the patient but will need to be treated if damaged.

14. B. The foramen ovale communicates with the infratemporal fossa but not directly with the pterygopalatine fossa. The other formina communicate with the pterygopalatine fossa.

15. C. Lemierre's syndrome is a disease usually caused by the bacterium Fusobacterium necrophorum. Typically this affects young, healthy adults. Infection leads to inflammation and thrombosis of the internal jugular vein. Septic emboli cause many of the resulting symptoms.

16. B. The major blood supply is typically from the ascending pharyngeal artery. Multiple small vessels may arise from the carotid artery.

17. B. From the upper incisors the typically the cricopharyngeus is at 15 cm, the aorta 22 cm, the left main bronchus 27 cm and the gastro-oesophageal junction at 38 cm.

18. D. Surgery has no place in the initial management of nasopharyngeal carcinoma, other than obtaining a tissue diagnosis. High dose radiotherapy to the primary site and both sides of the neck with or without chemotherapy is the primary treatment, even in the presence of lymph node metastasis. There is good evidence that chemo-radiotherapy produces better survival than radiotherapy alone, and is commonly used in advanced disease.

Surgery has a role in patients who relapse with lymph node metastasis following primary treatment.

19. C. Positron emission tomography is a non-invasive, diagnostic imaging technique for measuring metabolic activity of cells. The PET-FDG scan uses of a small amount of radioactive material, FDG (fluoro-deoxyglucose) which is concentrated in cells exhibiting high rates of glycolysis. The tracer is therefore not specific to cancer cells and can produce false positive results when concentrated in tissues that also exhibit high rates of glycolysis, such as inflammatory cells. The resolution of PET is being improved but requires a tumour load greater than a few cells. The advent of PET-CT has improved anatomical localization but not soft tissue resolution.

20. B. 75% of cases of medullary thyroid carcinoma are sporadic while the remaining are genetically determined. Phaeochromocytomas, frequently bilateral and multiple, occur in MEN IIA and IIB syndromes. Hyperparathyriodism due to multigland disease can develop in MEN IIA but is not seen in MEN IIB.

Characteristic phenotypic abnormalities are seen in MEN IIB and include mucosal neuromata and ganglioneuromas, marfanoid habitus, and cardiac abnormalities. Familial medullary thyroid carcinoma is not associated with endocrine abnormalities. The genetic basis of the familial tumours is missense germline mutations in the RET protooncogene.

21. C. The most common relationship is for the spinal accessory to be lateral to IJV at the skull base. Less commonly the spinal accessory nerve can emerge medial to the IJV and rarely the IJV can split around the nerve.

22. D. During sleep physiological muscle relaxation is maximal in REM sleep.

The multiple sleep latency test measures the time to fall asleep in a darkened room on several separate occasions across the day following an instruction to fall asleep. An average time of less than 7 minutes is considered to be evidence of pathological sleepiness.

Pulse oximetry is commonly used in the diagnostic testing for OSA. However, a normal oximetry tracing does not exclude OSA, particularly in younger patients who do not desaturate during their apnoea episodes

Continuous positive airway pressure (CPAP) has been established as the treatment of OSA.

See: Scottish Intercollegiate Guidelines Network. Management of obstructive sleep apnoea/hypopnoea syndrome in adults. 2003

23. D. There is limited evidence that UVPP has a beneficial role in OSA. Palatal surgery can make the subsequent use of continuous positive airway pressure (CPAP) more difficult and it is therefore not a first line intervention.

Several studies have demonstrated that the presence of OSA is an independent predictor of hypertension, allowing for other compounding factors.

Weight management is considered an important therapeutic treatment for all patients with snoring/OSA.

The DVLA requires that he cease driving. As he has a group 2 licence (HGV), driving will be permitted only when satisfactory control of his symptoms have been achieved and confirmed by a specialist.

Current evidence suggests the maximal benefit of treatment is in those patients with a RDI > 14 and that this can help reduce daytime sleepiness, quality of life, blood pressure and mood.

See: Scottish Intercollegiate Guidelines Network. Management of obstructive sleep apnoea/hypopnoea syndrome in adults. 2003

24. C. The initial FNA was reported as Thy 1 (non-diagnostic) and was therefore repeated. The second FNA was reported as Thy 3 (follicular lesion/suspected follicular neoplasm). The majority of patients with a Thy 3 FNA will require surgical removal of the lobe containing the nodule with completion thyroidectomy if malignancy is confirmed by histology. Occasionally an FNA is reported as Thy 3 due to some suspicious findings but may be Thy 2 or Thy 4. The text of the report should indicate these suspicious and the case discussed at the MDT.

MRI and CT scanning can be useful to delineate the size of the goitre. However, iodinated contrast media should be avoided as this reduces the subsequent radio-iodide uptake by thyroid tissue and therefore can limit the use of I^{131} post operatively.

Thyroglobulin is used in the surveillance of thyroid cancer following surgery. However the measurement of thyroglobulin before thyroidectomy has no diagnostic or prognostic value and therefore should not be requested.

25. E.   Although you will wish to drain the oedema, and some surgeons would advocate this as part of the procedure, the first priority should be to take biopsies of any suspicious areas to exclude malignancy.

26. B.   The fundamental frequency of a person's voice is a function of the mass per unit length and the tension in the vocal cords. If the mass per unit length increases, as in Reinke's oedema, the pitch drops. Drainage of Reinke's oedema is likely to result in a raising of fundamental frequency of the voice. It is particularly important to warn female patients that their voice may be unrecognisable from its former quality.

27. A.   The very minimum requirement for a voice clinic is the presence of an ENT surgeon and a speech and language therapist. In some voice clinics, a manual therapist may attend to address musculoskeletal tension issues, and a psychologist may help with the psychological aspects of dysphonia. A singing teacher may also be of great help in treating professional voice users.

28. D.   The corrected calcium is within normal limits. Therefore no further treatment is required. Hypocalcaemia causes neuromuscular and cardiac abnormalities. The patient may report perioral parasthesia and in severe cases demonstrate irritability, confusion, hallucinations or seizures.

Neurologic findings include Chvostek sign and Trousseau sign, facial tetany and carpopedal spasm respectively. On an ECG they may have cardiac dysrhythmias and a prolonged QT interval.

29. D.   Most tumours of the parapharyngeal space are metastatic disease or direct extension from adjacent spaces. Primary parapharyngeal space tumours are rare, with the majority being benign (80%). The majority of these are salivary gland neoplasia from the deep lobe of the parotid or minor salivary gland tumours.

The stylomandibular ligament separates the parapharyngeal space from the submandibular space.

The superior boarder of the parapharyngeal space is the temporal bone. The fascia connecting the medial pterygoid plate and the spine of the sphenoid passes medial to the foramen ovale and foramen spinosum and these are not considered part of the space.

The parapharyngeal space is divided into pre and post styloid spaces. The pre-styloid space contains the retromandibular portion of the deep lobe of the parotid, minor salivary glands, branches of the trigeminal nerve, the ascending pharyngeal artery and the pharyngeal venous plexus. The post-styloid space contains the internal carotid artery, internal jugular vein, cranial nerves IX–XII, cervical sympathetic chain, lymph nodes and glomus bodies.

30. B. The pre-epiglottic space is bounded anteriorly by the thyrohyoid ligament. The posterior boundary is the epiglottis.

31. B. Squamous cell carcinomas arising in the post-cricoid region are associated with iron deficiency anaemia (Kelly–Patterson Brown or Plummer–Vinson syndromes) and are more common in females.

The hypopharynx is divided into the posterior pharyngeal wall, post cricoid and pyriform sinus.

Pooling of saliva in the pyriform sinus (Chevalier–Jackson sign) is a sign of pathology in the pyriform sinus.

Direct spread of tumours in can occur through the aryepiglottic fold into the paraglottic space.

32. B. The original description of the vocal fold was by Hirano, who described five layers: the outer layer of squamous epithelium; the superficial lamina propria, which is also known as 'Reinke's space'; then the intermediate lamina propria, the deep lamina propria and the vocalis muscle.

Hirano M: Structure and vibratory behaviour of the vocal folds. Dynamic Aspects of Speech Production 1977; eds. 13–27

33. E. A well differentiated follicular thyroid cancer cannot be differentiated from a benign follicular lesion based on FNAC. Histological diagnosis is required to confirm the diagnosis and therefore most of these cases will require surgical removal of the implicated nodule and discussion at an MDT.

34. B. Orbital decompression is a recognized treatment for thyroid eye disease. Indications for treatment include visual loss due to compressive optic neuropathy, exophthalmos causing cosmetic changes and exposure keratitis. Diplopia occurring pre-operatively or post-operatively is relatively common and may necessitate ocular procedures.

35. A. Neck metastases from nasopharyngeal carcinoma are graded differently from other tumours:
- Nx: nodes cannot be assessed
- N0: no regional lymph node metastasis
- N1: Unilateral metastasis in lymph nodes < 6 cm above the supraclavicular fossa
- N2: Bilateral metastasis in lymph nodes < 6 cm above the supraclavicular fossa
- N3: a Metastasis in a lymph node(s)> 6 cm
  b extension to the supraclavicular fossa.

36. D. Thyroid tissue in a lymph node was previously referred to as a lateral aberrant thyroid. This is now recognized as being metastatic well-differentiated papillary thyroid cancer. As such, referral to the MDT and surgery will be required. Interpretation of the FNA is made in the context of accurate clinical information regarding the site and a good quality aspirate.

37. B. There is an elongated styloid process, also known as Eagle's syndrome. This can cause symptoms attributed to irritation of the glossopharyngeal, trigeminal, facial and vagus nerves. The symptoms include throat discomfort, a foreign body sensation and neck pain which may be worse on swallowing.

38. B. Location of parathyroid tissue commonly requires more than one modality. A sestamibi scan combined with ultrasound will commonly locate a parathyroid adenoma. Radio-iodine isotope scanning is used in the follow-up of thyroid malignancy, and has no role in parathyroid tumours.

39. C. Surgery is the mainstay of treatment for medullary thyroid cancer. Surgery in childhood is used to prophylactically remove the thyroid in those patients with multiple endocrine neoplasia syndrome. While radiotherapy has not been shown to improve survival it may be used to control local symptoms. Chemotherapy is generally considered ineffective but has been used for progressive symptoms. Radioactive iodine is not used.

See: Guidelines for the management of thyroid cancer. British Thyroid Association. 2002

40. E. Excision of a second branchial arch cleft is usually performed in a skin crease and may require a step incision to follow the tract. The greater auricular nerve is at risk during this incision. As subplatysmal flaps are raised it is possible to damage the marginal mandibular nerve. As the cyst is followed this may pass through the bifurcation of the carotid artery and superior laryngeal nerve, hypoglossal and glossopharyngeal nerves can be damaged.

41. D. In all but professional voice users, damage to the superior laryngeal nerve is asymptomatic. However, in singers or other performers, superior laryngeal nerve palsy can be devastating.

42. B. This is a T2 tumour because there is involvement of more than one subsite, but the tumour measures less than 4cm and there is no fixation of the hemi-larynx. The subsites of the hypopharynx are the postcricoid, the posterior pharyngeal wall, and the pyriform fossa.

T-staging of hypopharyngeal cancer:

- T1: Tumour limited to one subsite of hypopharynx and 2cm or less in greatest dimension
- T2: Tumour invades more than one subsite of hypopharynx or an adjacent site, or measures more than 2 cm but not more than 4 cm in greatest dimension, without fixation of hemilarynx
- T3: Tumour more than 4 cm in greatest dimension or with fixation of hemilarynx
- T4a: Tumour invades thyroid/cricoid cartilage, hyoid bone, thyroid gland, oesophagus, or central compartment structure (including strap muscles and subcutaneous fat)
- T4b: Tumour invades prevertebral fascia, encases carotid artery, or invades mediastinal structures

See also the Scottish Intercollegiate Guidelines Network (SIGN) guidelines on Diagnosis and management of head and neck cancer <www.sign.ac.uk>.

43. C. The incidence of papillary carcinoma arising in a thyroglossal duct cyst is < 1%. Fine needle aspiration cytology should suggest the diagnosis pre-operatively. If it is diagnosed post-operatively, the management should be as for any other well-differentiated thyroid cancer.

44. D. Post-operative radiotherapy should be given to any patient at high risk of locoregional recurrence. All of the above except D should ideally receive radiotherapy.

1 A 3-year-old child presents with a discharging sinus below the pinna. On closer inspection, you notice a sinus opening in the external auditory canal. What would be the next appropriate step?

   A Proceed to excision excising an ellipse of skin and removing the whole tract.
   B Arrange a fistulogram to assess the course of the fistula.
   C Arrange an ultrasound scan.
   D Refer the child to the paediatricians because he may have multiple anomalies.
   E Arrange an MRI scan.

2 Which of the following muscles is most important in opening of the eustachian tube?

   A Levator veli palatini
   B Tensor veli palatini
   C Salpingopharyngeus
   D Buccinator
   E Lateral pterygoid

3 A 6-month-old child is being followed up with laryngomalacia having being diagnosed following a microlaryngoscopy and bronchoscopy. In which of the following situations would you consider surgical intervention?

   A Noisy breathing during feeding
   B Cyanotic episodes
   C Failure to thrive
   D A and B
   E B or C

4   **You are called to see a 3-day-old baby born to a lady of Afro-Caribbean descent. The child was born full term in the breech position by vaginal delivery. The child has a firm palpable mass in the region of the right sternocleiodomastoid muscle. What is the MOST appropriate management?**

A   Fine needle aspiration cytology

B   Massage and observation

C   Surgical exploration

D   Commence anti-tuberculous therapy

E   Intralesional sceleroscent injections

5   **You are working in London and asked to consent a child born on 24 January 2004 for a tonsillectomy following persistent episodes of tonsillitis. His biological father accompanies him. The father informs you that he has a different surname from his son and has never been married to the child's mother although he is named on the birth certificate as the father. The father wants the operation to proceed. What is the MOST appropriate course of action?**

A   Inform the father that only the mother can consent for treatment and therefore postpone surgery.

B   Cancel surgery and see if the child has any further episodes of tonsillitis in the next 6 months.

C   Allow the father to sign the consent form and proceed with surgery.

D   Alter the order of the list so that the hospital lawyer can be contacted.

E   Get a colleague to witness the consent.

6   **Which of the following statements BEST describes the development of the ear in an otherwise healthy child?**

A   At birth the ossicles are approximately half their eventual adult size.

B   The auricle develops from the ectoderm of the first three branchial arches.

C   At birth the auricle is adult shape and size.

D   The first otologic structure to develop is the inner ear.

E   The bony labyrinth develops from six separate centres of ossification.

7 A child presents with a normal auricle, complete external
ear canal atresia and normal middle ear and ossicles. What
is the likely timing of the insult that would have caused these
changes?

A   0–15 weeks gestation

B   15–25 weeks gestation

C   25–40 weeks gestation

D   Post natal

E   It is not possible to predict the timing

8 A 3-year-old child (10 kg) presents to the Accident
and Emergency department with a post-tonsillectomy
haemorrhage. The child is crying, has a heart rate of
140 beats/minute and has a normal blood pressure
(110/60 mmHg). Up to what volume of blood are they
LIKELY to have lost?

A   50 ml

B   120 ml

C   175 ml

D   200 ml

E   235 ml

9 Which subtypes of human papillomatosis virus (HPV) are
associated with recurrent respiratory papillomatosis?

A   11 & 16

B   6 &16

C   6 & 11

D   16 & 18

E   6, 11, 16 & 18

10 Vaccination against the human papilloma virus (HPV) is
being introduced in to the UK to prevent cervical cancer.
The vaccine Gardasil (Sanofi Pasteur MSD) offers protection
against which strains of HPV?

A   11 & 16

B   6 &16

C   6 & 11

D   16 & 18

E   6, 11, 16 & 18

11 You are referred a child with congenital hearing loss and a goitre. A diagnosis of Pendred's syndrome is made. Which of the following statements is LEAST likely to be true?

A Pendred's is a common form of syndromal deafness.

B A CT scan of the auditory system may show a Mondini malformation.

C A CT scan of the auditory system may show a large vestibular aqueduct.

D Pendred's syndrome is diagnosed when there is a decrease in radioactive iodide discharge from the thyroid following the administration of potassium perchlorate.

E The chance of a further child being born to the same parents with the condition is 50%.

12 A 14-year-old boy presents to the hospital accompanied by his father with hypovolaemic shock and active bleeding following a secondary tonsillar haemorrhage. He has a haemoglobin of 5.5 g/dl on a blood gas. You advise that the boy requires resuscitation including blood transfusion and return to theatre to arrest the haemorrhage. The boy informs you that he is a Jehovah's Witness and he forbids you to perform a blood transfusion. What is the next MOST appropriate action?

A Call a senior colleague and ask him to come in to give a second opinion.

B Call the blood bank to find a cell saver device.

C Perform the blood transfusion as clinically indicated.

D Contact the hospital lawyer for advice.

E Perform all measures necessary except the transfusion.

13 A child's trachea is narrowed from its normal diameter of 8 mm to 4 mm. What effect is this likely to have on the airflow during quiet breathing?

A 4-fold increase in resistance

B 8-fold increase in resistance

C 12-fold increase in resistance

D 16-fold increase in resistance

E 256-fold increase in resistance

14 **What is the MOST common soft tissue malignancy in childhood?**

A Osteosarcoma

B Rhabdomyosarcoma

C Fibro-ossifying sarcoma

D Hemangiopericytoma

E Neurofibrosarcoma

15 **Which of the following statements concerning microtia is correct?**

A Bilateral microtia is more common than unilateral pathology.

B The auricle is formed from 1st branchial arch derivatives.

C The 6 hillocks of His form the auricle.

D The auricle is full-sized at birth.

E Surgery to repair the atretic ear canal is usually performed at the time of auricular reconstruction.

16 **A 4-year-old child presents with a rapidly enlarging right parotid mass, and facial palsy. Ultrasonography confirms an intraparotid mass. What is the MOST common malignant process in this situation?**

A Squamous cell carcinoma

B Lymphoma

C Mucoepidermoid carcinoma

D Rhabdomyosarcoma

E Adenoid cystic cell carcinoma

17 **Concerning Usher's syndrome, which of the following statements is FALSE?**

A If both parents are carriers of the defective gene the chance of having a child with the syndrome is 25%.

B Usher's syndrome type 1 is associated with reduced vestibular function.

C Usher's syndrome type 2 is less common than type 1.

D Retinitis pigmentosa results in blindness.

E Usher's syndrome type 1 is associated with a predominantly low tone hearing loss.

18 Concerning the development of the upper aerodigestive tract, which of the following statements is FALSE?

A The larynx develops in part from the 4th–6th branchial arches.

B At birth the larynx is higher in the neck than in the adult and descends through the first 2 decades of life.

C The laryngeal musculature develops in part from the 4th branchial arch.

D Laryngomalacia is the commonest cause of infantile stridor.

E Laryngomalacia is commoner in premature infants with neuromuscular immaturity.

19 Which of the following statements concerning cutaneous haemangiomas is true?

A Haemangiomas are considered vascular malformations.

B Haemangiomas are always present at birth.

C Surgical removal of a haemangiomas is the primary treatment.

D A port wine stain is a cutaneous haemangioma involving the face.

E Subglottic haemangiomas are frequently associated with cutaneous lesions.

20 In the Myer–Cotton grading of subglottic stenosis, a 60% stenosis would be…?

A Grade I

B Grade II

C Grade III

D Grade IV

E None of the above

21 Concerning choanal atresia, which of the following statements is true?

A It may be associated with genital defects

B Is always apparent at birth

C Is usually not apparent until teenage years

D Is usually bilateral

E Is more common in males

22 **Regarding tracheo-oesophageal fistula, which of the following statements is true?**

A It is more common in females.

B Type II is the most common type.

C It has an association with dystopia canthorum.

D It has a close association with vascular anomalies.

E It may be diagnosed on antenatal ultrasonography.

23 **A cutaneous capillary vascular malformation typically**

A Is not obvious at birth, but grows rapidly in the first year of life

B Involutes between the ages of 2 and 9 years

C Is more common in males

D May be associated with underlying meningeal vascular malformations

E Does not respond to laser therapy

24 **Which of the following is LEAST associated with Down's syndrome?**

A Low-set ears

B Subglottic stenosis

C Subglottic haemangioma

D Otitis media with effusion

E Relative IgA deficiency

25 **All of the following are associated with Gorlin's syndrome EXCEPT which?**

A Meningiomas

B Skin basal cell carcinomas

C Odontogenic keratocysts

D Choanal atresia

E Autosomal dominant inheritance

26 A child is undergoing a rigid bronchoscopy. During the procedure it is noted that the patient's right arm has become pale and pulseless. The arm becomes pink and with a good pulse on removal of the bronchoscope. Compression of which vessel is likely to be the cause of this phenomenon?

A Right common carotid artery

B Left common carotid artery

C Brachiocephalic artery

D Right subclavian vein

E Right vertebral artery

27 Bat ear deformities as a result of a lack of an anti-helical fold are due to abnormal development of which structure?

A 1st hillock of His

B 2nd hillock of His

C 3rd hillock of His

D 4th hillock of His

E 5th hillock of His

28 You are asked to see a 14-year-old girl with a 3-day history of a painful left neck. On examination she is diffusely tender along the sternocleidomastoid mastoid muscle but there is no focal mass. She has a low grade fever and a raised CRP (42) but is otherwise well. She is known to suffer from homocystinuria. From the history and examination what is the most likely diagnosis?

A Acute lymphoblastic leukaemia

B Internal jugular vein thrombosis

C Rhabdomyosarcoma

D Common carotid artery thrombosis

E Carotid body tumour

29 You are referred a 6-year-old boy with a history of a choking episode whilst playing two days ago. This is his chest X-ray:

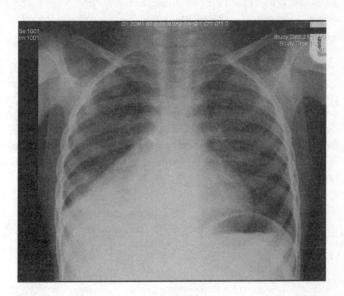

You plan to take him to the operating theatre. What would be the most appropriate method of induction of anaesthesia in this case?

A Rapid sequence induction and orotracheal intubation

B Propofol intravenous induction and orotracheal intubation

C Propofol intravenous induction and laryngeal mask airway placement

D Gas induction and naso-pharyngeal tube insertion

E Gas induction and orotracheal intubation

30 You are asked to see a 2-year-old child with suspected sinusitis. Which of the following sinuses is UNLIKELY to be involved?

A Sphenoid

B Ethmoid

C Maxillary

D All of the above: a child of this age would not develop sinusitis

E They all have an equal chance of being involved

31 **What is the most appropriate method of calculating the circulating blood volume of a 2-year-old child?**

A   5% of body weight

B   20% of body weight

C   20 ml/kg

D   40 ml/kg

E   80 ml/kg

32 **A mother attends the clinic with her 3-year-old son. She tells you that he has had 3 episodes of green rhinorrhoea in the last 18 months. Each of these has lasted 2 weeks, between times the child has been well and is healthy on examination. She is concerned about his immune status, what is the most appropriate course of action?**

A   Arrange immunoglobulin testing

B   Schedule the child for examination of the nose under anaesthetic and perform bilateral antral washouts (BAWO)

C   Prescribe a 2-month course of prophylactic low-dose antibiotics

D   Reassure the mother and discharge the child

E   Reassure the mother and review the child in 4 months

1. E. This is a first branchial cleft fistula (collaural fistula). These congenital fistulas can take a course close to the facial nerve. From the possible answers given, MRI is the most appropriate answer, although some surgeons would proceed to surgery directly, with identification of the facial nerve via a modified Blair ('lazy S') incision.

2. B. The Eustachian tube is normally closed. It is opened by contraction of the tensor veli palatini muscle.

3. E. Cyanotic episodes and failure to thrive suggest severe laryngomalacia. In these instances further intervention is indicated.

4. B. This is likely to be a haematoma of the sternocleiodomastoid muscle. Conservative and supportive measures are the most appropriate first stage of therapy.

5. C. The father has the legal responsibility for the child and can consent to the procedure.

Consent need only be given by one person with parental responsibility but is good practice to involve both parents.

The law in relation to parental responsibility has been revised. Originally those people with parental responsibility were described in the Children Act 1989. They included both the child's parents if they were married at the time of conception or birth or the child's mother if they were not married. Fathers not married to the mother could have acquired parental responsibility through a court order, subsequent agreement or marriage.

However, more recently the law has been changed to recognise unmarried fathers and so in relation to children born after 1 December 2003 (England and Wales), 15 April 2002 (Northern Ireland) or 4 May 2006 (Scotland), both of a child's legal parents have parental responsibility if they are registered on the child's birth certificate. This applies irrespective of whether the parents are married or not.

6. D. The inner ear develops first as the otic placode forms in week 3 of gestation and the semicircular canals are fully formed by week 8.

The ossicles are adult-sized at birth. The auricle develops from condensations of mesoderm of the first and second branchial arches. These give rise to the six hillocks of His. At birth the auricle is adult-shaped but is not adult-sized until approximately 9 years.

The bony labyrinth develops from 14 centres of ossification.

7. C. Auricular formation occurs in the first trimester. By week 12 the auricle is formed by fusion of the hillocks of His and is adult-shaped by week 20. Formation of the middle ear begins at week 10 and the ossicles are adult-sized by 16 weeks. The external ear canal develops from the ectoderm of first pharyngeal groove. This forms a solid core which does not hollow out until week 28.

8. B. This child is in type I shock (up to 15% blood volume loss). The circulating volume of a child is approximately 80ml/kg. Therefore the child has lost up to 120mls of blood.

9. C. HPV subtypes 6 and 11 are associated with recurrent respiratory papillomatosis and are also associated with genital warts. HPV types 16 and 18 have most often been associated with cancer in the genital area.

10. E. Gardasil HPV vaccine protection against HPV strains 6, 11, 16 and 18.

11. E. Pendred's syndrome is the most common syndromal form of deafness and is associated with developmental abnormalities of the cochlea, sensorineural hearing loss, and goitre.

Pendred's syndrome is associated with temporal bone abnormalities ranging from a large vestibular aqueduct to the Mondini malformation. It is inherited in an autosomal recessive pattern of inheritance so that the chance of a subsequent child with the condition is 1 in 4.

The condition is caused by a defect in the organification of iodine. The perchlorate test is used in the diagnosis of Pendred's syndrome. The test is performed by administering radiolabelled iodine and measuring the radioactivity emitted from the thyroid. Potassium perchlorate is then administered. This is a competitive inhibitor of iodide transport into the thyroid. The emittance of radioactivity is again measured over the thyroid and compared to initial result.

In unaffected individuals, the amount of radiolabelled iodine in the thyroid remains stable due to the rapid oxidation of iodide to iodine and its subsequent incorporation into thyroglobulin.

In affected individuals the transport of iodine is delayed, resulting in iodide passing into the blood. This manifests as a decrease in radiolabelled iodine in the thyroid.

12. C. An adult Jehovah's Witness can refuse a blood transfusion. However, a minor cannot refuse a transfusion if it is required for a life-saving procedure, even if deemed competent.

13. D. This relates to Poiseuille's Law, which states that resistance to airflow is inversely proportional to the fourth power of the airway radius when laminar flow is present. Therefore if the radius is halved, without altering the length or viscosity then the resistance increases 16-fold.

14. B. Rhabdomyosarcoma is the most common soft tissue malignancy in childhood and occurs most commonly in the head and neck.

15. C. The majority of cases of microtia are unilateral (90%). The auricle is formed from the 6 hillocks of His, three from each of the 1st and 2nd branchial arches, and at birth the auricle is approximately 65% of adult size.

Surgery to the atretic ear canal is controversial and in a unilateral microtia with contralateral normal hearing is not usually undertaken due to the poor results, as middle ear abnormalities are associated with microtia.

16. C. Mucoepidermoid carcinoma is the commonest malignant salivary gland tumour in children. Most are low grade and have a good prognosis.

17. E. Usher's syndrome is inherited in an autosomal recessive pattern. Type 1 is the commonest and associated with profound congenital deafness, abnormal vestibular function and retinitis pigmentosa occurring in the first decade of life.

Type 2 is associated with a moderate to severe congenital deafness, normal vestibular function and retinitis pigmentosa occurring in the second or third decade of life.

18. E. The exact aetiology of laryngomalacia is unknown but it is not commoner in premature infants.

19. E. Up to 50% of patients with a subglottic haemangioma will have a cutaneous lesion. However, of those patients with a cutaneous lesion only a small percentage will have a subglottic haemangioma.

Haemangiomas are benign vascular tumours that appear after birth, while vascular malformations are present at birth. In general, surgery is reserved for those tumours not responding to either conservative treatment with observation, steroids, or laser ablation, or which are in a position to cause problems such as to the eye.

A port wine stain is a cutaneous capillary vascular malformation.

20. B. The Myer–Cotton grading system describes the percentage of tracheal stenosis.
- Grade I: 0–50%
- Grade II: 51–70%
- Grade III: 71–99%
- Grade IV: complete obstruction

Stridor at rest occurs in stenoses of approximately grade III and above.

21. A. Choanal atresia may be seen as part of the CHARGE (Colomba, Heart defects, Atresia choanae, Retarded growth, Genital defects, Ear anomalies) syndrome, or with Treacher–Collins syndrome. Unilateral atresia which is most common may not present until later in childhood. It is more common in females.

22. E. Tracheo-oesophageal fistula are more common in males and Type I is the most common. There is only rarely an association with vascular anomalies. Impairment of fetal swallowing may lead to polyhydramnios on ultrasound.
Dystopia canthorum is associated with Waardenburg's syndrome.

23. D. Vascular malformations are typically visible at birth, but may be difficult to find and whereas cutaneous haemangiomas involute between 2 and 9 years of age, vascular malformations do not. There is equal incidence in males and females.
The Surge–Weber syndrome consists of a cutaneous capillary vascular malformation and an underlying intracranial vascular malformation.
Cutaneous capillary vascular malformations typically do respond to laser therapy, particularly pulsed dye lasers and argon lasers.

24. C. Down's syndrome is associated with increased risk of all of the above except subglottic haemangioma. The relative IgA deficiency predisposes these children to upper respiratory tract infections.

25. D. Gorlin's syndrome (Gorlin–Goliz syndrome) is associated with:
- multiple basal cell carcinomas
- cutaneous abnormalities
- skeletal anomalies
- cranial calcifications
- multiple odontogenic keratocysts.

26. C. The right arm is supplied with blood by the right subclavian artery, a branch of the brachiocephalic artery, which often passes obliquely across the trachea and may become compressed during brochoscopy.

27. D. The auricle develops from the 6 hillock of His. The first three from the first branchial arch and the latter three from the second. The first three hillocks form the tragus, helical crus and helix. The fourth hillock forms the antihelix, the fifth the scapha and the sixth the lobule.

28. B. Homocystinuria is an inherited autosomal recessive disorder of methionine metabolism. This causes a widespread disorder of the connective tissue, muscles, CNS, and cardiovascular system, often with a marfanoid appearance.

   Thrombotic complications are common affecting the venous and arterial vasculature. These complications often result in death before the age of 30. From the clinical scenario described it is likely that the child would be more unwell if thrombosis of the common carotid artery had occurred.

29. D. This child requires rigid bronchoscopy to retrieve the pin in the right main bronchus. This is best achieved by performing a gas induction and placing a naso-pharyngeal tube, allowing the child to breathe spontaneously while the procedure is performed.

30. A. The development of the sinuses proceeds as follows:
• Maxillary sinuses are present at birth.
• Ethmoid sinuses are present at birth.
• Sphenoid sinus pneumatization starts in the third year of life.
• Frontal sinuses are not present at birth and are not aerated before 6 years of age.

31. E. The circulating volume of a child is 8–9% of body weight, or 80ml/kg. The hourly fluid maintenance for a child is:
• 4 ml/kg for the first 10kg
• then add 2 ml/kg for the next 10kg
• then add 1 ml/kg for any weight after 20kg.

Example: a 25 kg child requires:

• 4 ml × 10 kg = 40
• Plus 2 ml × 10 kg = 20
• Plus 1 ml × 5 kg = 5
• Total: 40 + 20 + 5 = 65 ml/hr
   A child in shock should receive a fluid challenge of 20 ml/kg of crystalloid. A further 2 fluid challenge boluses of 20 ml/kg may be given if the child does not respond.

32. D. It is not unusual for a healthy child to have at least 3 upper respiratory tract infections per year. No specific investigations are required and the mother should be reassured.

1 A 42-year-old male presents with nasal obstruction. A CT of the paranasal sinuses is reported as showing opacification of the right maxillary sinus with 'double density' signals throughout the sinus. Which of the following is the LEAST likely pathology?

A Allergic fungal sinusitis

B Chondrosarcoma

C Inverted papilloma

D Antrochoanal polyp

E Ossifying fibroma

2 Concerning nasal ciliary physiology and anatomy, which of the following statements is LEAST accurate?

A The nose is lined by ciliated pseudostratified glandular columnar epithelium.

B The nasal cilia are arranged as 9 microtubule doublets formed in an outer circle around a central pair.

C The outer microtubular doublets are linked by the protein nexin.

D Ciliary movement is described as having 2 phases.

E Normal ciliary beat frequency is approximately 10–25 beats per minute.

3 Which of the following bones is LEAST likely to be transected as part of an endoscopic transethmoidal sphenoidotomy?

A Uncinate process

B Bulla ethmoidalis

C Anterior wall of the sphenoid

D Palatine bone

E Ground lamella of the middle turbinate

4   When performing an external ethmoidectomy, at what distance from the anterior lacrimal crest are you most likely to find the posterior ethmoidal artery?

A   12 mm

B   24 mm

C   30 mm

D   36 mm

E   42 mm

5   Which of the following bones do not form part of the osteology of the lateral nasal wall?

A   Maxilla

B   Palatine

C   Ethmoid

D   Perpendicular plate of the sphenoid

E   Inferior turbinate

6   In a 70 kg male being prepared for a lymph node biopsy under local anaesthetic. What is the maximum volume of 2% lidocaine without adrenaline that can be injected?

A   5 ml

B   10 ml

C   15 ml

D   20 ml

E   25 ml

7   Ohngren's line is used as a prognostic indicator in management of carcinoma of the maxillary sinus. This line is described as an imaginary plane perpendicular to the intersection between…?

A   The lateral canthus and the angle of the jaw

B   The lateral canthus and the menton

C   The medial canthus and the angle of the jaw

D   The tragus and the nasal tip

E   The tragus and the menton

8   **Performing FES surgery you are operating to remove the anterior ethmoidal air cells when you see clear fluid flowing from the region of the lateral lamella of the cribiform plate. What is the next most appropriate action?**

   A   Stop surgery, wake the patient up and see if the clear fluid continues.
   B   Inject intrathecal fluorscein to confirm the presence of a CSF leak.
   C   Perform a local repair of the probable CSF leak.
   D   Continue the surgery, then pack the nose with a nasal tampon for 48hours.
   E   Request the neurosurgeons to perform a craniotomy and dural repair.

9   **A 14-year-old boy presents with a unilateral nasal mass. A coronal STRI image from the MRI is shown. The lesion fills the nasal cavity and involves the pterygopalatine fossa. What is the most appropriate management plan?**

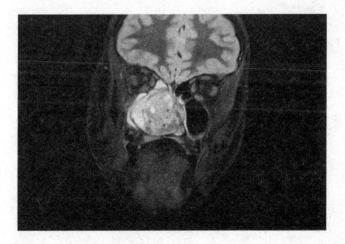

   A   Observe with serial MRI scans
   B   Arrange external beam radiotherapy
   C   Perform a biopsy to confirm the diagnosis
   D   Arrange for surgery to be performed
   E   Arrange arterial embolization.

10 A 46-year-old man presents with a exophytic tumour arising from his right maxillary antrum extending onto the hard palate and anterior maxillary wall only. It has not invaded the orbital walls or involved his subcutaneous tissues. A biopsy is reported as squamous cell carcinoma. According the TNM classification what stage would this tumour be?

    A T1
    B T2
    C T3
    D T4a
    E T4b

11 You wish to use a urinary catheter as a post nasal pack in a patient with epistaxis. The only available size is a French size 24. What is the diameter of the tube?

    A 4 mm
    B 6 mm
    C 8 mm
    D 10 mm
    E 12 mm

12 Which of the following does not form part of the bony orbital cavity?

    A Lacrimal bone
    B Zygomatic bone
    C Palatine bone
    D Greater wing of the sphenoid
    E Nasal bone

13 A patient presents with CSF rhinorrhoea. What are the likely signal characteristics of CSF on MR imaging?

    A High intensity signal on T1-weighted imaging
    B Low intensity signal on T2-weighted imaging
    C High intensity signal on T2-weighted imaging
    D Enhancement following administration of gadolinium
    E MRI poorly identifies CSF

14 Which of the following statements best describes Wegner's
    granulomatosis?

    A Untreated, the disease is usually asymptomatic for many years.
    B Cirrhosis of the liver is a common feature of the disease.
    C The perinuclear anti-neutrophil cytoplasmic antibody (p-ANCA)
       is highly sensitive for the disease.
    D Is most common in those of Afro-Caribbean origin.
    E The cytoplasmic anti-neutrophil cytolpasmic antibody (c-ANCA)
       is highly sensitive for the disease.

15 A 44 year male with a 4-month history of anosmia reports
    that he can still smell ammonia. Which cranial nerve is likely
    to be responsible for this?

    A One – olfactory
    B Five – trigeminal
    C Seven – facial
    D Nine – glossopharyngeal
    E Ten – vagus

16 Concerning the embryology of the nose and paranasal sinuses
    which of the following statements is FALSE?

    A The frontal sinus originates from pneumatization of the frontal recess
       and is usually not visible at birth.
    B At 2 years of age the floor of the maxillary sinus is usually higher than
       the floor of the nasal cavity.
    C Failure of resorption of the naso-buccal membrane results in choanal
       atresia.
    D An absence of nasal bones on intra uterine screening is associated with
       Down's syndrome.
    E Branchio-oto-renal syndrome is characterized by abnormal cilia function
       and chronic sinusitis.

17 According to the Lund & Mackay grading system for sinus opacification, what would be the score for this CT of the paranasal sinuses?

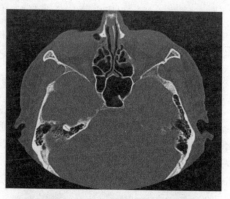

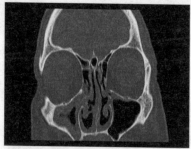

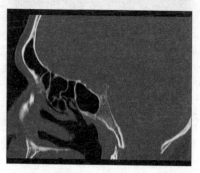

A   Zero
B   Two
C   Six
D   Eight
E   Ten

**18   A 60-year-old man is referred by his GP with unilateral
      nasal obstruction. The GP has organized for him to have a
      CT scan before the appointment. The most appropriate next
      investigation would be:**

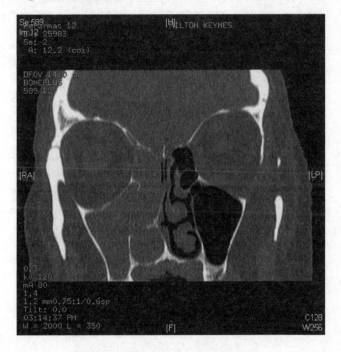

A   Referral to the head & neck multidisciplinary team
B   Referral to the specialist rhinologist in your hospital
C   Schedule the patient for endoscopic sinus surgery
D   Schedule the patient for biopsy
E   Arrange an MRI of the neck to examine nodal status

19 Which of the following is **NOT** closely related to the frontal recess?

A Agger nasi
B Ethmoidal bulla
C Middle turbinate
D Lamina papyracea
E Superior turbinate

20 A 79-year-old man presents to the clinic with left-sided nasal discharge and obstruction. A mass is found arising from the ethmoid sinuses and histology shows an adenocarcinoma. Which of the following is the most significant risk factor for developing this disease?

A Smoking
B Alcohol
C A and B
D Wood dust
E Asbestos

21 Which of the following is **LEAST** likely to improve the symptoms from an anterior nasal septal perforation?

A Nasal hygiene
B Free tissue transfer cartilage graft repair (cartilage, perichondrium only)
C Silastic button placement
D Local flap repair
E Free tissue transfer composite graft repair (epithelium, cartilage, epithelium)

1. D. Allergic fungal sinusitis is characterized by areas of increased attenuation on non-contrast CT. These hyperdense and heterogenous densities in an opacified sinus are also referred to as the 'double density' sign and most likely represent higher levels of magnesium, manganese, and iron in fungal mucin. The double density sign is also seen in chondorsarcoma, inverted papilloma, and ossifying fibroma.

2. E. Normal ciliary beat frequency is approximately 1000–1500 beats per minute.

The epithelium lining of the upper airways is with ciliated pseudostratified glandular columnar epithelium. There is a 9+2 arrangement of the normal cilia, with 2 central microtubules surrounded by 9 microtubule doublets. Nexin arms link the outer doublets. Ciliary movement has an effective stroke phase that sweeps forward and a recovery phase during which the cilia bend backward and extend into the starting position for the stroke phase.

3. D. A endoscopic transethmoidal sphenoidotomy involves an uncinectomy, anterior and posterior ethmoidectomy before opening the face of the sphenoid infero-medially.

4. D. From the anterior lacrimal crest the anterior ethmoidal artery is approximately 24 mm. The posterior ethmoidal artery is a further 12 mm and the optic nerve a further 6 mm.

5. D. The lateral nasal wall is formed by the bones of the maxilla, palatine, ethmoid, lacrimal, and inferior turbinate.

6. C. The maximum dose of lidocaine without adrenaline is 3–5 mg/kg up to 200 mg. The maximum dose for a 70 kg male is theoretically 350 mg. A solution of 2% lidocaine contains 20 mg/ml.

7. C. Ohngren's line is between the medial canthus and the angle of the jaw. Tumours above this line are associated with a worse prognosis than those below the line.

8. C. In this situation were a CSF leak is highly likely and this is noted at the time of surgery, closure at the primary surgery should be performed. Fluorescein, while used to help with the identification of a CSF leak, is not licensed for this. The consent process should take account of this.

9. D. This is likely to represent a juvenile nasopharyngeal angiofibroma. These are highly vascular benign tumours and therefore a biopsy is not appropriate. Surgery is the treatment of choice and radiotherapy is generally only used for very extensive lesions that cannot be removed surgically or for recurrent disease. Embolization of the sphenopalatine artery may be appropriate.

10. B. Maxillary sinus TNM Classification (AJCC)
Primary tumour (T)
- T1: Tumour limited to the antral mucosa with no erosion or destruction of bone
- T2: Tumour causing bony erosion or destruction including extension to hard palate and/or middle meatus, except extension to posterior antral wall or pterygoid plates
- T3: Tumour invading any of: posterior antral wall, subcutaneous tissues, floor or medial orbit wall, pterygoid fossa, ethmoid sinuses
- T4a: Tumour invades anterior orbital contents, skin of cheek, pterygoid plates, infratemporal fossa, cribiform plate, sphenoid or frontal sinuses
- T4b: Tumour invades any of: orbital apex, dura, brain, middle cranial fossa, cranial nerves other than V(b), nasopharynx, and/or clivus

11. C. The French catheter scale is used to measure the outside circumference. The diameter (mm) can be calculated by dividing the French size by Pi. Therefore a French size 24 equals a diameter of 8 mm.

12. E. 7 bones are considered to make up the bony orbital cavity. The frontal, Zygomatic, Maxillary, Lacrimal, Palatine, ethmoid and sphenoid (greater and lesser wings).

13. C. CSF has a high intensity signal on T2-weighted imaging and a low intensity signal on T1-weighted images.

14. E. Wegner's is characterized by necrotizing granulomas involving the upper respiratory tract; vasculitis of small- and medium-sized vessels and glomerulonephritis. Untreated, the disease carries a very poor prognosis. The c-ANCA is more than 90% sensitive and specific for the disease, while 20–40% of cases have raised p-ANCA.

15. B.   The trigeminal nerve supplies innervation to the nose and is sensitive to noxious chemical stimuli, such as ammonia.

16. E.   Branchio-oto-renal syndrome is characterized by abnormalities of the ear, branchial clefts, and renal dysplasia.

The frontal sinus originates from pneumatization of the frontal recess into the frontal bone, and is not usually visible at birth. It is usually complete by the age of 20.

The maxillary sinus undergoes two periods of rapid growth associated with dental development (3 years and 7–12 years). Initially the floor of the sinus is above that of the nasal floor, but later it is below the nasal floor.

Prenatal markers for Down's syndrome include absent or hypoplastic nasal bones.

Abnormal cilia function is seen in Kartagener's syndrome and primary ciliary dyskinesia.

17. C.   The Lund & Mackay score is calculated by scoring each sinus complex (maxillary, anterior ethmoids, posterior ethmoids, frontal and sphenoid sinus) 0–2, where 0=absence, 1=partial, 2=complete opacification. The osteomeatal complex is scored (0= clear or 2=obstructed). A maximum score of 24 is possible.

This series of scans is scored as: right anterior ethmoids = 1; right maxillary sinus = 1; right osteomeatal complex = 2 and left osteomeatal complex = 2 each. Total 6.

18. D.   This unilateral expansile but not erosive mass probably represents an inverted papilloma. It is important initially to establish the diagnosis and then to plan definitive treatment.

19. E.   The boundaries of the frontal recess are as follows:
• medially – middle turbinate
• laterally – lamina papyracea
• superiorly – frontal sinus drainage pathway
• posteriorly – ethmoid bulla
• anteriorly – agger nasi

20. D.   Hard wood dust is a recognized risk factor for the development of adenocarcinoma of the ethmoid sinuses. The link was first made in High Wycombe, where there was a large number of workers in the furniture industry.

21. B.   Asymptomatic nasal septal perforations may simply require nasal hygiene. A large perforation (> 2 cm) that causes subjective nasal obstruction, or one which whistles or bleeds, can often be managed with placement of a silastic button. Smaller symptomatic perforations may be amenable to surgical closure with a composite graft of cartilage, perichondrium and skin, harvested from the pinna.

1　A 4-year-old child has sustained a clean facial laceration which requires closure. Which of the following is the most acceptable form of closure?

A　5/0 silk

B　2/0 undyed vicryl

C　4/0 Monocryl

D　Skin clips

E　4/0 dyed vicryl subcuticular

2　Concerning rhinoplasty techniques, which of the following techniques is UNLIKELY to achieve the stated aim.

A　An onlay graft overlying the alar domes will increase tip projection.

B　Separating the medial crura of the lower lateral cartilages from the septum will decrease tip projection.

C　Removing part of the cranial edge of the lower lateral cartilage 'cephalic shave' will cause caudal tip rotation.

D　Using the lateral crura of the lower lateral cartilages to elongate the medial crura 'lateral crural steel' will increase tip projection.

E　Interdomal sutures will increase tip projection.

3　Concerning facial aesthetic analysis, which of the following statements is FALSE?

A　The width of the eye is approximately one fifth the width of the face.

B　The nasolabial angle describes the nasal projection in relation to the upper lip.

C　The nasolabial angle is more obtuse in Caucasian women then men.

D　A tip projection ratio of 0.6 is ideal (tip projection ratio: radix-tip distance/tip to alar cheek junction distance).

E　The hair line to alar base distance represents approximately two thirds of the facial height.

4   **Concerning melanoma, which of the following statements is LEAST likely to be true?**

A   Tumour thickness and ulceration are the most important histological markers of prognosis.

B   Superficial spreading melanoma has an initial radial growth phase followed by a vertical growth phase.

C   Nodular melanomas are less aggressive than other forms of melanoma.

D   Xeroderma pigmentosa represents an inherited risk of developing melanoma.

E   Fitzpatrick type I skin carries a higher risk of developing melanoma than type VI skin.

5   **Which of the following are not used in the AJCC staging system for melanoma?**

A   Tumour thickness

B   Tumour ulceration

C   Size of lymph nodes

D   Number of lymph nodes

E   Sentinel node biopsy results

6   **The nose is subdivided into how many aesthetic subunits?**

A   5

B   7

C   8

D   9

E   11

7   **A patient suffers a knife wound to the face. The wound is closed primarily, tension-free and forms a well-healed scar. The patient wishes to know how strong the tissue is compared to normal skin. Which answer is most appropriate?**

A   Compared to normal skin the tissue is 10% as strong.

B   Compared to normal skin the tissue is 30% as strong.

C   Compared to normal skin the tissue is 50% as strong.

D   Compared to normal skin the tissue is 80% as strong.

E   Compared to normal skin the tissue is 100% as strong.

8   **Which of the following represent the lowest risk of developing a basal cell carcinoma?**

A   Basal cell nevus syndrome (Gorlin's syndrome)

B   Sun exposure

C   Xeroderma pigmentosa

D   Immunosupression

E   Fitzpatrick skin type 5

9   **A Z-plasty is used on a patient. The advantages include all of the following except…?**

A   Excision of the scar

B   Shortening of the scar

C   Lengthening of the scar

D   Reorientation of the scar

E   Release tension on the scar

10   **The sural nerve can be used as an interposition cable graft in facial nerve repair. Which of the following statements is FALSE?**

A   The nerve is found approximately 1 cm posterior to the lateral malleolus.

B   Sectioning the nerve will leave result in parasthesia along the lateral aspect of the foot.

C   The nerve contains mixed sensory and motor innervation to the flexor digiti minimi brevis.

D   Up to 40 cm of the nerve can be harvested.

E   It is in close approximation to the short saphenous vein.

11   **In normal wound healing when would you expect the number of fibroblasts to peak?**

A   Within 6 hours

B   Within 24 hours

C   Within 3 days

D   Between 3 and 5 days

E   Between 6 and 7 days

12   **The following diagram represents a rhomboid rotational flap.
Which of the following statements is correct?**

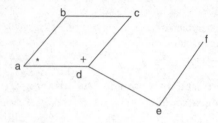

A   When closing a rhomboid flap point d is transposed to point a

B   Angle * is 80 degrees

C   Angle + is 150 degrees

D   Up to 4 separate flaps could be raised

E   The distance from point c to point f should be as small as possible when using this flap on the face.

13   **Tumours of the lower lip are typically:**

A   Basal cell carcinomas

B   Associated with poor oral hygiene

C   Associated with neck metastases in 45% of patients at presentation

D   Almost universally in males

E   Associated with late metastasis in 50%

14   **Which of the following would be the LEAST appropriate
recipient site for a full-thickness skin graft?**

A   Pericranium

B   Muscle

C   Fat

D   Cartilage

E   Bone

15   **Which of the following flaps relies on the principle of delayed
division of the pedicle?**

A   Duformentel flap

B   Abbe flap

C   Karapandzic flap

D   Gillies fan flap

E   Radial forearm flap

16 **Concerning reconstructive flaps, which of the following are incorrectly matched?**

A Latissimus dorsi flap is based on the thoracodorsal artery

B Pectoralis major flap is based on the thoracoacromial artery

C Sternocleidomastoid flap is based on the ascending pharyngeal artery

D Deltopectoral flap is based on the perforating branches of the internal thoracic artery

E Midline forehead flap is based on the supratrochlear artery

17 **Following excision of a 4 mm diameter BCC from the tip of the nose with a 3 mm margin, which of the following is the LEAST appropriate method of repair?**

A The use of a full-thickness skin graft 'Wolfe graft' using post auricular skin

B The use of a nasolabial advancement flap based on the facial artery

C Primary closure

D The use of a paramedian rotational forehead flap based on the supratrochlear artery

E The use of a bilobed rotation flap

18 **A 65-year-old man presents with a basal cell carcinoma of the lower lip. You decide to resect the lesion and reconstruct using an Abbe flap. Which of the following statements regarding the flap is INCORRECT?**

A The Abbe flap is generally used when the lip defect involves one third to two thirds of the lip.

B The Abbe flap is generally not used when the defect involves the commisure.

C The Abbe flap can be based on the superior or inferior labial artery.

D The labial artery is a branch of the facial artery and lies deep to the obicularis oculi muscle.

E The Abbe flap is a single stage procedure.

19 Concerning reconstructive flaps, which of the following can be considered INCORRECT?

A A full thickness skin graft contains the epidermis and the whole of the dermis.

B A full thickness skin graft will usually give a better cosmetic result than a split skin graft.

C Most local skin flaps on the face are random pattern flaps deriving their blood supply from the dermal-subdermal plexus.

D With a local advancement flap Burrows triangles may allow the flap to sit better.

E A ratio of 1:2 pedicle width to flap length should be strictly adhered to on the face.

20 The diagram shows the planning for a bilobed (Zitelli) flap to be used on the dorsum of the nose. Which of the following statements is FALSE?

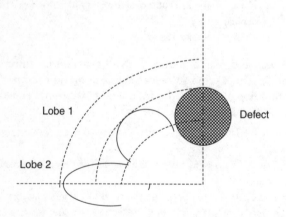

A The maximal angle of rotation is 90–100 degrees.

B The width of lobe 1 should be the same width as the defect.

C When using this to reconstruct defects on the nose there is a random pattern blood supply.

D The most tension when closing is usually found in the defect site.

E A disadvantage of the flap is a complex scar.

21 **In which of the following situations would Moh's micrographic surgery be least appropriate?**

A A large squamous cell carcinoma on the cheek

B A recurrent squamous cell carcinoma on the forehead

C Age > 80

D Cosmetically sensitive area

E A basal cell carcinoma arising in the posterior triangle of the neck

22 **A 75-year-old man is undergoing a local anaesthetic excision of a suspected basal cell carcinoma on his cheek. What clinical margin of excision is most appropriate?**

A 0 mm

B 2 mm

C 5 mm

D 1 cm

E 2–3 cm

1. C.   Undyed vicryl might be acceptable, but 2/0 is far too large a suture material in a child's skin. Of the above, Monocryl, an absorbable monofilament material, would give the most acceptable result.

2. C.   Performing a 'cephalic shave' will cause cranial tip rotation.

3. B.   The nasolabial angle describes the angle between the lip and the caudal end of the nose. This angle describes the degree of nasal tip rotation. The width of the eye is approximately one fifth of the facial width and is equal to the alar base width and intercanthal distance.

   The nasolabial angle is 95–110 degrees in women and 90–95 degrees in men.

   Tip projection can be calculated as the ratio of the radix-tip distance tip and the alar-cheek junction distance. In an aesthetically balanced face this ratio is approximately 0.6.

   The face is divided into thirds by horizontal lines drawn adjacent to the menton, alar base, brows and hairline.

4. C.   Nodular melanomas demonstrate predominantly a vertical growth and therefore are considered aggressive.

   Tumour thickness, as defined by the Breslow depth, is the most important histological determinant of prognosis. Ulceration is also important and its presence leads to upstaging of the disease.

   Superficial spreading melanoma does have an initial radial growth phase followed by a vertical growth phase.

   Xeroderma pigmentosa and dysplastic nevus syndrome represent congenital risk factors for developing skin cancers.

   Fitzpatrick classified skin types such that type I never tans and always burns. This represents a higher risk than those skins that always tan and never burn.

5. C.   The AJCC (American Joint Committee on Cancer, 2002) uses tumour thickness to stage melanoma. The 2002 AJCC modifications also include histological ulceration and the number of lymph nodes involved rather than size.

   Microscopic regional lymph node metastasis as detected by sentinel lymph node biopsy differentiate tumours into those with micro or macroscopic nodal metastasis.

6. D. The nose has been divided into aesthetic subunits. There are paired lateral nasal wall units, paired alar units, paired soft tissue triangles and single dorsum, tip, columella subunits.

Burget GC, Menick FJ. Subunit principle in nasal reconstruction. *Plast Reconstr Surg* 1985; **76**: 239–47

7. D. A scar that has healed correctly is expected to attain 80% strength compared to normal tissues.

8. E. All of the other answers are associated with an increased risk of developing BCC. Fitzpatrick classified skin types such that type 1 is fair skin and type 6 is black skin. The latter represents a lower risk of developing skin cancer.

9. B. A Z-plasty is used to excise a scar, reorientating and lengthening a scar. The angle subtended by the arms dictates the lengthening that can be expected.

10. C. The sural nerve has the advantage over the great auricular nerve of having greater length (up to 40 cm) as well as a greater number of neural fascicles. The nerve contains only sensory fibres and lateral foot numbness results after sectioning.

The sural nerve is located between the lateral malleolus and the Achilles tendon, lying deep to the short saphenous vein.

The flexor digiti minimi brevis is supplied by the superficial branch of the lateral plantar nerve.

11. E. During the proliferative phase of wound healing fibroblasts are attracted by chemotactic factors and begin to arrive on day 3, and peak by day 7.

12. D.

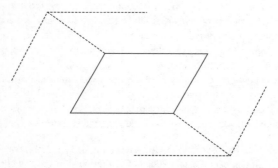

Up to 4 flaps can be designed. Angle * is 60 degrees and angle + 120 degrees. Point d closes to point b. This is a random pattern flap so therefore it is important to consider the distance c to f as the flap receives its blood supply from this pedicle.

13. D. Tumours of the lower lip are squamous cell carcinomas in 98% of cases. There is an overwhelming preponderance of males (ratio 80:1) over females. Clinically apparent cervical metastases are seen in fewer than 10% of patients. Around 5–15% of patients will develop lymph node metastases at some time in the future.

14. E. A full-thickness skin graft relies on its new site for a blood supply. Therefore, any of the above except bare bone would suffice as a recipient site.

15. B. The Abbe lip switch flap is usually used to transfer tissue from the lower to the upper lip. A wedge excision of the upper lip tumour is performed. A wedge of the lower lip is taken, but not completely excised, as the inferior labial artery blood supply is preserved. The lower lip flap is then rotated into the upper lip defect. Three weeks later, the pedicle is divided and the suturing completed.

    A Duformental flap is similar to a rhomboid flap.

    A Karapandzic flap is a bilateral advancement flap extending onto the cheek for lip tumours.

    Gillies fan flap is a large rotation flap used for lip tumours.

    A radial forearm flap is a free-tissue transfer involving a microvascular anastomosis.

16. C. The sternocleidomastoid flap is a random pattern flap and receives a segmental blood supply from the transverse cervical artery, the superior thyroid artery and the occipital artery.

17. C. The defect described would have a diameter of 10 mm. Due to the limited quantity and mobility of the skin on the tip of the nose primary closure is not appropriate. The other methods would be suitable.

18. E. The Abbe flap can be used for defects of the upper or lower lip involving between one third and two thirds of the lip. The flap is a two stage procedure based on the labial artery with division of the pedicle at 2–3 weeks.

19. E. In general a ratio of 1:2–3 pedicle width to flap length is advised. However, on the face this can often be increased to 1:4–5 due to the excellent blood supply.

    A full thickness skin graft (FTSG) contains the epidermis and the whole of the dermis in contrast to split thickness skin graft that contains the epidermis and less than the whole of the dermis. FTSGs do give better cosmetic results.

20. D. The bilobed flap can be used on the nose and exploits the greater skin laxity in other areas to move skin in. The usual angle of rotation is 90–100 degrees. Lobe 1 is usually the width of the defect while lobe 2 is usually narrower. The flap is a stepwise rotational flap. The first lobe should be closed under no tension. The most tension on the wound will be involved in closing the defect formed from lobe 2. The scar is generally complex when closed and this may be a disadvantage cosmetically.

21. E. Moh's micrographic surgery refers to complete micrographic excision of the tumour using intra-operative histopathology to assess for positive margins. This technique is particularly useful for:
- recurrent tumours
- tumours measuring > 2 cm
- those with an aggressive histology and
- those in cosmetically sensitive areas, since wide excision is often difficult.

22. B. For basal cell carcinoma, a 2–3 mm margin will assure histopathologic clearance in 95% of cases.

Tio core guidelines:

    Hi Risk BCC : 4mm margin

    Low Risk BCC : 3mm margin.

EXTENDED MATCHING ITEMS (EMIs)

1 A Schwanoma
   B Paraganglioma
   C Fibrosarcoma
   D Wegner's
   E Sarcoidosis
   F Chordoma

For each of the following questions, select the most likely histological diagnosis. Each response may be used once, more than once, or not at all.

1 Following excision of a neck mass the histology reports a cellular pattern of compact spindle cells (Antoni type A) with more loosely arranged hypocellular zones surrounding it (Antoni B).

2 Following excision of a posterior pharyngeal wall lesion the histology is reported as showing chronic inflammation, necrosis, granulomas with multinucleated giant cells, vasculitis, and microabscesses.

3 Following a post nasal space biopsy a histopathological report of physaliferous cells with a 'soap bubble' appearance and compressed nuclei.

4 Following a biopsy of neck mass the report is of a tumour composed of cell nests or 'zellballen' surrounded by sustentacular cells.

2 A Radicular cyst
    B Ossifying fibroma
    C Fibrous dysplasia
    D Odontogenic keratocyst
    E Ameloblastoma
    F Brown tumour
    G Odontogenic myoxoma
    H Cementoblastoma
    I Central giant cell granuloma
    J Metastatic tumour

For each of the following questions, select the most likely diagnosis. Each response may be used once, more than once, or not at all.

1 A 15-year-old patient presents with a history of multiple basal cell carcinomas. Which odotogenic lesion should be suspected?

2 A 75-year-old patient is found to have a lesion in her mandible. Biochemical investigations reveal a serum corrected calcium of 3.05 mmol/l (2.12–2.62), phosphate 0.78 mmol/l (0.8–1.45) and PTH 262 ng/l (12–72) What is the likely diagnosis?

3 A 14-year-old girl who is under the care of the paediatricians for precocious puberty presents with a unilateral bony swelling over the maxilla. What is the most likely diagnosis?

3   A   Schwartze sign (reddish hue of the tympanic membrane)

B   Brown's sign (blanching of the tympanic membrane on pneumatic otoscopy)

C   Hennebert's sign (ocular deviation with pneumatic otoscopy)

D   Paracusis Willisii (apparent improvement in hearing for conversation against background noise)

E   Diplacusis (apparent difference in pitch of a tone perceived by both ears)

F   Oscillopsia

G   Brun's sign (intermittent headache, vertigo and vomiting)

H   Hitselberger's sign (reduced sensitivity over the postero-superior aspect of the concha)

I   Griesinger's sign (oedema and tenderness over the mastoid cortex)

For each of the following diagnoses, select the most likely sign. Each response may be used once, more than once, or not at all.

1   Which sign is likely to be positive in a patient diagnosed with otosyphilis?

2   Which sign may be positive in a patient with pulsatile tinnitus?

3   Which sign may be present in a patient with an acoustic neuroma?

4   A   Cytomegalovirus

B   Rubella

C   Mumps

D   Parvovirus

E   Measles

F   Toxoplasmosis

G   Treponema pallidum

H   Norwalk virus

I   Varicella zoster

J   Herpes simplex

For each of the following questions, select the most likely syndrome from the list above. Each response may be used once, more than once, or not at all.

1   Which infection is commonest cause of infective congenital sensorineural hearing loss?

2   Which infection is most commonly associated with unilateral sensorineural hearing loss acquired in childhood?

3   Which infection has been implicated in the aetiology of otosclerosis

5   A   Apert syndrome

B   Alport syndrome

C   Crouzon syndrome

D   Treacher–Collins syndrome

E   Pfeiffer syndrome

F   Saethre–Chotzen syndrome

G   Jackson–Weiss syndrome

In each of the following questions, select the most likely syndrome. Each response may be used once, more than once, or not at all.

1   Which syndrome exhibits autosomal dominant inheritance and often results in brachycephaly, midfacial hypoplasia, and normal intelligence?

2   Which syndrome exhibits autosomal dominant inheritance and often results in auricular malformations, conductive hearing loss and normal intelligence?

3   Which syndrome is associated in males with progressive SNHL, haematuria, and chronic renal failure?

6   A   Foramen ovale

B   Foramen rotundum

C   Superior orbital fissure

D   Inferior orbital fissure

E   Internal acoustic meatus

F   Foramen magnum

G   Jugular foramen

H   Pterygoid canal (vidian canal)

I   Hypoglossal canal

J   Petrotympanic fissure (Glaserian fissure)

K   Foramen spinosum

L   Olfactory groove

Select the correct foramen for each of the following structures. Each response may be used once, more than once, or not at all.

1   The spinal accessory nerve exits through it.

2   The lesser petrosal nerve exits through it.

3   The chorda tympani enters the infratemporal fossa through it.

7 A Bells palsy
   B Millard–Gubler syndrome
   C Mobius syndrome
   D Ramsey Hunt syndrome
   E Melkerson–Rosenthal syndrome
   F Diabetus mellitus
   G Guillain–Barré syndrome
   H Lyme disease
   I Botulism
   J Syphilis
   K HIV
   L Sickle cell disease
   M Von Recklinghausen's disease

For each of the following situations, select the most likely diagnosis. Each response may be used once, more than once, or not at all.

1 A 45-year-old female presents with a severe headache, onset bilateral facial nerve palsy (House–Brackmann grade III) of 3 days duration and a swollen lip. The remainder of the examination was normal.

2 A previously fit and well 45-year-old woman presents a two week history of shortness of breath and bilateral facial palsy occurring over the preceding 12 hours. On examination she has generalized motor weakness and shallow respirations.

3 A 4-year-old child presents with a 3 day history of a left facial nerve palsy, an excoriated region on the left forehead with surrounding erythema, having recently returned from visiting relatives in Australia. The rest of the examination was normal.

8 A Deltopectoral flap
   B Midline forehead flap
   C Temporalis flap
   D Pectoralis major flap
   E Latissimus dorsi flap
   F Trapezius flap
   G Sternocleidomastoid flap
   H Radial forearm flap
   I Scapular flap
   J Rectus abdominus flap
   K Lateral thigh flap

From the above list, select the correct flap. Each response may be used once, more than once, or not at all.

1 A fasciocutaneous flap based on the first four perforating branches of the internal mammary artery.
2 Which flap receives a segmental blood supply which includes the transverse cervical artery?
3 Which flap is unlikely to be available in a patient with Poland's syndrome?

9 A Suprabullar recess
   B Hiatus semilunaris
   C Agger nasi cell
   D Bulla ethmoidalis
   E Kuhn cell
   F Haller cell
   G Uncinate process
   H Frontal process of the maxilla
   I Middle meatus
   J Inferior meatus
   K Superior meatus
   L Supreme meatus
   M Sphenoethmoidal cell (Onodi)

Select the correct anatomical structure based on the following descriptions. Each response may be used once, more than once, or not at all.

1 Two dimensional space lying between the bulla and the uncinate process.
2 Anterior wall of the frontal recess.
3 Embryologically derived from the 2nd basal lamella.

10 A Apoptosis
    B Mitosis
    C Meiosis
    D Exon
    E Intron
    F Codon
    G Gene
    H Genome
    I Messenger RNA
    J Oncogene
    K Transcription factor
    L RNA interference

From the list above, select the correct response to the following questions. Each response may be used once, more than once, or not at all.

1 The end of which mechanism results in cell death?
2 What is the name given to the total DNA contained in each cell?
3 A normally occurring mechanism for the cell to silence specific gene function?

11 A RNA interference
    B Northern blotting
    C Southern blotting
    D Western blotting
    E cDNA microarray
    F Polymerase chain reaction
    G Immunohistochemistry
    H Cell viability assay

For each of the questions below, select the correct technique from the list above. Each response may be used once, more than once, or not at all.

1 A technique for identifying a specific protein in a cell lysate.
2 A technique that can assess the expression of many thousands of genes using single strand oligonucleotides of known sequence.
3 A technique for amplifying DNA.

12 A Ménière's disease

   B Syphilis

   C Cogan's syndrome

   D Acoustic neuroma

   E Polyarteritis nodosa

   F Rheumatoid arthritis

   G Behçet's syndrome

   H Systemic lupus erythematosus

   I Wegener's granulomatosis

   J Sarcoidosis

Select the condition from the list above that matches each of the descriptions below. Each response may be used once, more than once, or not at all.

1 An autoimmune condition associated with ocular inflammation?

2 Associated with progressive sensorineural hearing loss and genital ulceration?

3 A condition that may be diagnosed by dark field microscopy?

13 A Atrophy

   B Dysplasia

   C Hamartoma

   D Hyperplasia

   E Hypertrophy

   F Metaplasia

   G Metastasis

   H Pleomorphism

For each of the questions below, select the correct physiological or pathological process from the list above. Each response may be used once, more than once, or not at all.

1 An increase in the number of cells per unit of tissue?

2 A change of one fully differentiated cell into another?

3 An increase in the size of individual cells?

14 A Polyglycolic acid (eg Vicryl)
    B Polydioxanone (eg PDS)
    C Polycaprone glycolide (eg Monocryl)
    D Polypropylene (eg Prolene)
    E Silk
    F Braided polyester (eg Ethibond)
    G Stainless steel

For each of the questions below, select the most likely suture material. Each response may be used once, more than once, or not at all.

1 Induces a local fibrotic reaction, and is degraded by proteolysis over a number of years.

2 An example of a synthetic monofilament that maintains tensile strength for many years.

15 A [Bracket open to the right
    B]   Bracket open to the left
    C △   Triangle
    D ○   Circle, unfilled
    E ●   Circle, filled
    F ↘   Arrow
    G ⌊
    H ⌋

For each of the questions below, select the correct audiological symbol from the list above. Each response may be used once, more than once, or not at all.

1 According to the British Society of Audiology, which symbol represents unmasked bone conduction?

2 According to the British Society of Audiology, which symbol represents left-sided uncomfortable loudness levels?

3 According to the British Society of Audiology, which symbol represents right air conduction?

16 A Fibroblast growth factor receptor 1
    B Fibroblast growth factor receptor 2
    C Fibroblast growth factor receptor 3
    D Fibroblast growth factor receptor 4
    E Collagen type 1
    F Collagen type 2
    G Collagen type 3
    H Collagen type 4

Select the correct responses from the list above. Each response may be used once, more than once, or not at all.

1 Achondroplasia is associated with a mutation in which gene?
2 Crouzon's syndrome is associated with a mutation in which gene?
3 Apert's syndrome is associated with a mutation in which gene?

17 A Acromegaly
    B Acrocephaly
    C Brachycephaly
    D Colpocephaly
    E Lissencephaly
    F Microcephaly
    G Plagiocephaly
    H Scaphocephaly
    I Trigonocephaly

Select the correct response for the questions below. Each response may be used once, more than once, or not at all.

1 Premature fusion of the coronal suture results in which abnormality?
2 What is the most common craniofacial abnormality found in Apert's syndrome?
3 Which craniofacial abnormality is most common?

18 A 5-year-old boy presents to the Accident and Emergency department with noisy breathing.

A Flexible nasendoscopy

B Immediate tracheostomy

C Laryngoscopy and intubation in the operating theatre

D Examination of the mouth

E Chest X-ray

F Soft tissue X-ray of the neck

G Rigid bronchoscopy

H CT scan of the neck

To obtain a diagnosis, which management would be most appropriate in the following situations? Each response may be used once, more than once, or not at all.

1 The child is febrile, tachycardic, drooling and has marked odynophagia

2 The child may have inhaled a foreign body

3 The child has been stridulous for many months

4 The child was diagnosed with tonsillitis 2 days ago

19 A child is found, at his neonatal screening test, to have a severe sensorineural hearing loss.

A Pendred's syndrome

B Usher's syndrome

C Waardenburg syndrome

D Alport syndrome

E Branchio-oto-renal syndrome

F Neurofibromatosis type II

G Jervell–Lange–Neilsen syndrome

H Treacher–Collins syndrome

I Stickler syndrome

Which of these syndromes would most likely apply in the following situations? Each response may be used once, more than once, or not at all.

1 The child has widely-spaced eyes

2 The child has Hirschprung's disease

3 The child has retinal flecks

4 The child has a goitre

5 The child as a prolonged QT interval on the ECG

20 A Vidian nerve
   B Facial nerve
   C Greater superficial petrosal nerve
   D Lingual nerve
   E Hypoglossal nerve
   F Descendens hypoglossi nerve
   G Lesser petrosal nerve

For each of the following questions select the correct nerve. Each response may be used once, more than once, or not at all.

1 Supplies only parasympathetic innervation to the nose
2 Contributes to the ansa cervicalis
3 Supplies parasympathetic innervation to the parotid gland
4 Is the continuation of Jacobsen's nerve
5 Is a branch of the glossopharyngeal nerve

21 Types of study:

   A Case-control study
   B Cohort study
   C Randomized controlled trial
   D Systematic review
   E Case series study

Which of type of study is best described in the following? Each response may be used once, more than once, or not at all.

1 A prospective comparison of two treatments
2 A retrospective study of patients with a disease in an attempt to identify risk factors for that disease
3 A survey to examine the prevalence of a disease
4 A prospective study in which subjects, initially disease-free, are followed up

22 Levels of evidence:

A Level 1a

B Level 1b

C Level 1c

D Level 2a

E Level 2b

F Level 2c

G Level 3a

H Level 3b

I Level 4

J Level 5

What level of evidence is seen in the following types of research? Each response may be used once, more than once, or not at all.

1 Individual RCT

2 Case series

3 Systematic review (with homogeneity) of randomized controlled trials

4 Expert opinion

23 A Behind-the-ear (BTE)

B Bone-conduction hearing aid

C Bone-anchored hearing aid (BAHA)

D In-the-ear (ITE)

E Vented mould behind-the-ear

F Body-worn hearing aid

G Cochlear implant

For each of the following situations, select the most appropriate initial hearing aid. Each response may be used once, more than once, or not at all.

1 A child of 5 years of age with a profound bilateral hearing loss

2 An adult with Down's syndrome with persistently discharging ears and a conductive hearing loss

3 An 80-year-old lady with severe rheumatoid arthritis who lives alone

4 A 30-year-old solicitor with a mild low-tone sensorineural hearing loss.

24 A 1 ml

B 3 ml

C 25 ml

D 50 ml

E 45 ml

F 90 ml

G 150 ml

In an average adult male patient, what is the maximum permissible volume for each of the following drug preparations? Each response may be used once, more than once, or not at all.

1 0.5% bupivacaine with adrenaline

2 0.25% bupivacaine with adrenaline

3 Dental Xylocaine®

4 25% cocaine paste

5 10% cocaine solution

25 A Dexamethasone, neomycin, acetic acid

B Dexamethasone, framycetin, gramicidin

C Hydrocortisone, gentamicin

D Triamcinolone, gramicidin, neomycin, nystatin

E Hydrocortisone, neomycin, polymixin B

F Clotrimazole

What active ingredients are in the following ear medications? Each response may be used once, more than once, or not at all.

1 Otosporin

2 Tri-adcortyl otic

3 Sofradex

4 Otomize

5 Canesten

26 A   Mucoepidermoid carcinoma

   B   Carcinoma ex-pleomorphic adenoma

   C   Adenocarcinoma

   D   Adenoid cystic carcinoma

   E   Acinic cell carcinoma

   F   Squamous cell carcinoma

   G   Basaloid carcinoma

   H   Rhabdomyosarcoma

For each of the following clinical scenarios, select the most likely diagnosis. Each response may be used once, more than once, or not at all.

1   A 45-year-old woman with a firm lesion on the hard palate and lung metastases.

2   A 70-year-old man with a longstanding parotid mass that then begins to enlarge rapidly

3   A 67-year-old smoker with a firm lesion on his lower lip

4   A 50-year-old woman with salivary gland malignancy and trigeminal symptoms

27 A   Chi-square test

   B   Student's t-test

   C   Mann–Whitney U test

   D   McNemar's test

   E   Spearman rank correlation

   F   Logistic regression

   G   Kruskal–Wallis test

What is the most appropriate statistical test in the following circumstances? Each response may be used once, more than once, or not at all.

1   Input variable and outcome variable are both ordinal

2   Input variable is nominal and outcome variable is non-normal

3   Input variable is nominal and outcome variable is normal

4   Input variable is nominal and outcome variable is quantitative discrete

28 A Standard deviation

    B Standard error of the mean

    C Type I error

    D Type II error

    E 95% Confidence Interval

    F Reference range

    G Standard error

For each of the following questions, select the correct statistical description. Each response may be used once, more than once, or not at all.

1 The sample mean plus or minus 1.96 times its standard error

2 Standard deviation/$\sqrt{n}$

3 An estimate of variability of observations

4 A measure of precision of an estimate of a population parameter

29 A Autosomal dominant

    B Autosomal recessive

    C X-linked

    D Usually sporadic

    E Variable penetrance

    F Imprinting

    G Variable expressivity

For each of the following conditions, select the most appropriate description. Each response may be used once, more than once, or not at all.

1 Waardenburg's syndrome

2 Alport syndrome

3 Usher's syndrome

4 Apert's syndrome

5 van der Woude syndrome

30 Branches of the external carotid artery

A Ascending pharyngeal
B Superior thyroid
C Lingual
D Facial
E Occipital
F Posterior auricular
G Superficial temporal
H Maxillary

For each of the following statements, select the correct artery. Each response may be used once, more than once, or not at all.

1 Winds around the body of the mandible
2 Passes through the pterygopalatine fossa
3 Is the dominant blood supply to a pharyngeal pouch
4 Is the origin of the superior labial artery
5 Is routinely ligated as part of a laryngectomy

31
A Polymyositis
B Scleroderma
C Achalasia
D Ganglionic degeneration
E Carcinoma
F Pharyngeal pouch
G Barrett's oesophagus

For each of the following situations, select the most likely diagnosis. Each response may be used once, more than once, or not at all.

1 Chagas disease
2 Aperistalsis, oesophageal dilatation and failure of relaxation of the lower oesophageal sphincter
3 Irregular appearance on contrast swallow
4 May be associated with Raynaud's phenomenon

32 A Pseudostratified ciliated columnar epithelium

     B Stratified squamous epithelium

     C Keratinized squamous epithelium

     D Pavement epithelium without cilia

     E Pseudostratified ciliated columnar epithelium with goblet cells

     F Pseudostratified non-keratinized stratified squamous epithelium

Match each of the anatomical locations with its correct epithelial type. Each response may be used once, more than once, or not at all.

1 True vocal cords

2 False cords

3 Mastoid antrum

4 Skin of pinna

5 Trachea

33 A Clotting screen

     B APTT

     C Bleeding time

     D Factor assays

     E Genetic screening

     F Platelet count

     G A and F

     H None of the above

For each of the clinical scenarios described, select the most appropriate blood test. Each response may be used once, more than once, or not at all.

1 A child due to undergo a tonsillectomy with a history of easy bruising and prolonged bleeding from trivial cuts

2 A 55-year-old man, otherwise in good health, admitted to hospital with an uncomplicated nosebleed (first episode) controlled by packing

3 A patient on intravenous heparin for a vascular procedure who develops a profuse nosebleed

4 An alcoholic man admitted with a nosebleed that is slow to respond to first aid

34 A Pemphigus
   B Pemphigoid
   C Candida
   D Leukoplakia
   E Erythroplakia
   F Lichen planus
   G Stevens–Johnson syndrome
   H Behçet's disease

Which of the above conditions is described in the following questions? Each response may be used once, more than once, or not at all.

1 A high propensity to undergo malignant degeneration
2 An idiosyncratic drug reaction
3 Seen in conjunction with arthritis, eye pain and genital ulcers
4 Due to IgG autoantibodies targeted against desmosomal components
5 Associated with skin 'target lesions'

35 A Lower lateral cartilage
   B Upper lateral cartilage
   C Nasal bones
   D Septal cartilage
   E Vomer
   F Perpendicular plate of ethmoid

For each of the questions below, select the correct answer from above. Each response may be used once, more than once, or not at all.

1 In order to achieve upward tip rotation in rhinoplasty surgery, which structure may be trimmed cephalically?
2 Which structure contributes most to columella show?
3 Which structure is most likely to be damaged during the incisions in an open rhinoplasty?

36 A Polysomnogram

B Overnight oxygen saturation monitoring

C Proceed direct to adenotonsillectomy

D Genetic screening

E X-ray of post-nasal space

F Sleep nasendoscopy

For each of the following clinical situations, select the most appropriate management of the patient. Each response may be used once, more than once, or not at all.

1 In clear-cut cases of obstructive sleep apnoea in a child of 5 years

2 When central apnoea is suspected

3 When OSA may be suspected in a child, but the clinical situation suggests that this may not be the case (for example if the child has small tonsils, and/or if the child is breathing freely through the nose)

37 A KTP

B CO_2

C Pulsed dye

D Holmium

E Argon

F Helium-Neon

For each of the following questions, select the correct type of laser from the list above. Each response may be used once, more than once, or not at all.

1 The laser with a depth of penetration of 0.3mm

2 The laser type used to give a 'targeting beam'

3 The laser used in dermatological conditions of the face

38 You are required to perform rigid bronchoscopy in an adult
who has inhaled a peanut. The scrub nurse is having some
difficulty assembling the instruments.

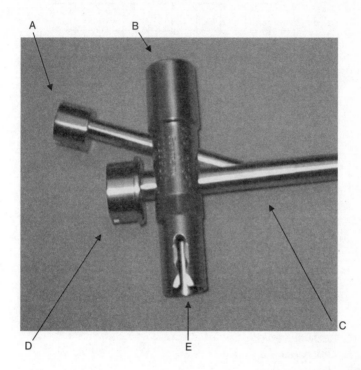

Correctly identify the following parts of the bronchoscope. Each response
may be used once, more than once, or not at all.

1 Connection to anaesthetic tubing
2 Suction port
3 Connection to light source

39 Examine the following trace of an auditory brainstem response (ABR).

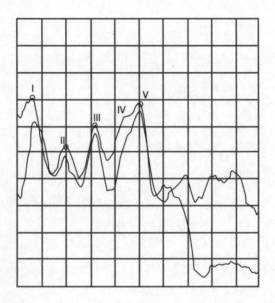

A Cochlea

B Cochlear nerve

C Cochlear nucleus

D Olivary complex

E Lateral lemniscus

F Corona radiata

G Auditory cortex

H Inferior colliculus

For each of the following questions, select the correct structure that is responsible for each peak on the ABR trace. Each response may be used once, more than once, or not at all.

1 Wave III

2 Wave IV

3 Wave V

4 Wave I

1

1.A. The histological pattern of alternating regions containing compact spindle cells Antoni type A with more loosely arranged Antoni type regions is characteristic of Schwanomas.

2.D. This histopathological description is characteristic of Wegner's.

3.F. A chordoma is a tumour of the notochord remnant.

4.B.

2

1.D. Gorlin's syndrome is a rare autosomal dominant condition associated with numerous pathologies including multiple basal cell carcinomas, odontogenic keratocysts, palmar or plantar pits, and bifid, fused, or markedly splayed ribs.

2.F. The patient has primary hyperparathyroidism. Brown tumors (osteoclastomas) are highly characteristic of primary hyperparathyroidism although they may also occur in secondary hyperparathyroidism as well. Brown tumors appear as single or multiple well-circumscribed lesions located within the facial bones as well as the hands, pelvis, and ribs.

3.C. Fibrous dysplasia presents as a painless bony enlargement and is characterized by a ground-glass radiographic pattern. There are two forms. The monostotic form is most common and frequently occurs in the jaws and cranium. The polyostotic form of the disease may be associated with McCune–Albright's syndrome (cutaneous pigmentation, autonomic hyper-functioning endocrine glands, and precocious puberty).

3

1. C. Hennebert's sign (ocular deviation with pneumatic otoscopy). This may also be positive in a patient with superior semicircular canal dehiscence. It is thought to be due to a fibrous band between saccule or utricle resulting in vestibular stimulation with footplate movement and greater with negative pressure.

2. B. Brown's sign (blanching of the tympanic membrane on pneumatic otoscopy) is seen in those patients with a glomus tympanicum tumour.

3. H. Hitselberger's sign. Due to a pressure effect on the facial nerve in the IAM.

4

1. A. Cytomegalovirus is the commonest cause of congenital hearing loss.

2. C. Hearing loss from mumps is acquired in childhood. It tends to occur after an episode of parotitis and is usually unilateral and may be profound.

3. E. Measles virus has been associated with otosclerotic foci and remains a possible aetiological factor in the development of the disease.

5

1. C. Crouzon syndrome is inherited in an autosomal dominant pattern and results in abnormalities of skull due to premature fusion of cranial sutures. The coronal and sagittal sutures most commonly involved. Other associated features include midface hypoplasia, exorbitism, lue ear, a high arched palate and normal intelligence.

2. D. Treacher–Collins syndrome exhibits autosomal dominant inheritance with complete penetrance and variable expression, up to 60% of cases are spontaneous new mutations. Features of the condition include maxillary hypoplasia, down sloping palpebral fissures and 'parrot face' appearance. Patients frequently have microtia or atresia with a predominantly conductive hearing loss. Most patients have normal intelligence.

3. B. This condition is inherited in an X-linked or autosomal dominant fashion is associated with progressive SNHL, nephritis, haematuria and chronic renal failure.

6

1. G.   The accessory nerve (or spinal accessory nerve) is the eleventh cranial nerve. It leaves the cranium through the jugular foramen along with the glossopharyngeal nerve (IX) and vagus nerve (X). There are two parts to the nerve. The spinal accessory nerve originates from neuronal cell bodies located in the cervical spinal cord and caudal medulla. Most are located in the spinal cord and ascend through the foramen magnum and exit the cranium through the jugular foramen. They are motor in function and innervate the sternocleidomastoid and trapezius muscles. The cranial root of the accessory nerve originates from cells located in the caudal medulla. They are found in the nucleus ambiguus and leave the brainstem with the fibres of the vagus nerve. They join the spinal root to exit the jugular foramen. They rejoin the vagus nerve and are distributed with the vagus nerve.

2. A.   The lesser petrosal nerve carries preganglionic parasympathetic fibres from the inferior salivary nucleus via the otic ganglion to innervate the parotid gland. It is derived from the facial and glossopharyngeal nerve via the tympanic plexus and passes through the foramen ovale to synapse in the otic ganglion. Postsynaptic fibres leave the otic ganglion, join the auriculotemporal nerve, and innervate the parotid gland.

3. J.   The chorda tympani, a branch of the facial nerve, carries special sensory fibers providing taste sensation from the anterior two-thirds of the tongue and presynaptic parasympathetic fibers to the submandibular ganglion, providing secretomotor innervation to two salivary glands: the submandibular gland and sublingual gland. The chorda tympani branches from the facial nerve, crosses the tympanic membrane and exits through the petrotympanic fissure into the infratemporal fossa. It then joins the lingual nerve (V3) and supplies preganglionic parasympathetic fibres to the submandibular and sublingual salivary glands via the submandibular ganglion. Special sensory (taste) fibres from the chorda tympani supply the anterior 2/3rds of the tongue via the lingual nerve.

7

1. E. Melkerson–Rosenthal Syndrome: The syndrome can present at any age, often with a history of recurrent symptoms that fluctuate in intensity. It is a syndrome consisting of the triad of recurrent lip oedema, recurrent facial paralysis and a fissured tongue. The changes involved in the lip include episodic non-tender lip swelling which may ultimately become rubbery hard (cheilitis granulomatosa). Only approximately one third of patients have recurrent facial nerve palsy as part of their syndrome and patients may not present with the complete triad. Other symptoms that may occur include headache, granular cheilitis, trigeminal neuraligia, dysphagia and laryngospasm.

2. G. Guillain–Barré syndrome (GBS) is a polyneuropathy affecting the peripheral nervous system, usually triggered by an acute infectious process. The disease is characterized by weakness and paresthesia affecting the lower limbs first, and progressing in an ascending fashion. The lower cranial nerves may be affected, leading to bulbar weakness

3. H. Lyme disease: Infection with the spirochete Borrelia burgdorferi results in Lyme disease. This tick-borne infection is endemic in certain regions of the USA as well as Europe and Australia. Facial palsy can occur with infection. Diagnosis is based on serological testing and the treatment is antibiotic therapy.

8

1. A. Deltopectoral.

2. G. Sternocleidomastoid receives a segmental blood supply from the occipital artery, superior thyroid artery, and the transverse cervical artery.

3. D. Poland's syndrome consists of unilateral absence or hypoplasia of the pectoralis muscle, most frequently involving the sternocostal portion of the pectoralis major muscle, and a variable degree of ipsilateral hand and digit anomalies, including symbrachydactyly.

9

1. B. The hiatus semilunaris is a two dimensional space lying between the bulla and the uncinate process. It is the common drainage site of the maxillary antrum, and anterior ethmoid sinuses.

2. C. Agger nasi cell. This is the most anterior pneumatized cell and is anterior to the vertical attachment of the middle turbinate. It forms the anterior boundary of the frontal recess.

3. D. Bulla ethmoidalis.

10

1. A.   Apoptosis is the process of programmed cell death. It is one of the main types of programmed cell death, and involves a series of programmed events.

2. H.   Genome.

3. L.   RNA interference is the mechanism by which small double-stranded RNAs can interfere with expression of any mRNA having a similar sequence. The RNAi effect has been exploited by molecular biologists to examining the role of those mRNA messages by their absence.

11

1. D.   Western blotting. This technique is used for analyzing mixtures of proteins to show the presence, size and abundance of one particular type of protein.

2. E.   cDNA microarray. Gene microarray technology has developed with the ability to deposit up to tens of thousands of single stranded DNA oligonucleotides on a single 'chip'. The different DNA fragments, arranged in such a way that the identity of each fragment is known through its location on the chip, allows the measurement of mRNA expression by hybridizing labelled cDNA to the chip

3. F.   PCR is a technique for replicating a specific piece of DNA in-vitro.

12

1. C.   Cogan's syndrome is thought to be an autoimmune disorder associated with aural symptoms of hearing loss, vertigo and tinnitus, and ocular inflammation

2. G.   Behçet's syndrome. An autoimmune condition with a triad of oral and genital ulcers, iritis or uveitis, and progressive hearing loss.

3. B.   Syphilis. Dark field microscopy involves a special microscope to examine a sample of fluid or tissue from an open sore (chancre) for the spyrochetes. If syphilis is present, it can be seen as corkscrew-shaped objects on the microscope slide. This test is used mainly to diagnose syphilis in an early stage.

13

    1. D.   Hyperplasia

    2. F.   Metaplasia

    3. E.   Hypertrophy

14

    1. E.   Silk is spun by silkworms. Over time the suture becomes absorbed by proteolysis over a number of years. Silk sutures excite an acute inflammatory reaction which leads to encapsulation by fibrous connective tissue.

    2. D.   Polypropylene (eg Prolene). This monofilament suture is biologically inert, eliciting minimal tissue reaction. It can maintain tensile strength for up to 2 years.

15

    1. C.   △

    2. G.   ⌐

    3. D.   ○

16

    1. C.   Fibroblast growth factor receptor 3

    2. B.   Fibroblast growth factor receptor 2

    3. B.   Fibroblast growth factor receptor 2

17

    1. C.   Brachycephaly

    2. C.   Brachycephaly. Bicoronal synostosis resulting in brachycephaly is the suture fusion found most often in Apert's and Crouzon's syndromes.

    3. H.   Premature fusion of the sagittal suture is the most common, resulting in scaphocephaly.
    The frequency of occurrence of the various types of craniosynostosis in the population is approximately as follows:
- sagittal 50–58%
- coronal 20–29%
- metopic 4–10%
- lambdoid 2–4%

18

1. C. This symptom complex suggests epiglottitis, and the child should be transferred immediately to theatre for intubation.

2. G. The most reliable way of making a diagnosis in this situation is to perform rigid bronchoscopy.

3. A. Flexible nasendoscopy is likely to suggest a diagnosis in this instance; he/she may have laryngeal papillomatosis or a laryngeal haemangioma.

4. D. A simple examination of the tonsils with a tongue depressor will confirm the diagnosis.

19

1. C. Along with abnormal pigmentation of iris, hair and skin, Waardenburg's syndrome is associated with dystopia canthorum (widely-spaced medial canthi) and Hirschprung's disease.

2. C.

3. D. Alport syndrome is associated with progressive renal failure and retinal flecks.

4. A. Pendred's syndrome is associated with goitre (usually evident before puberty) that results in hypothyroidism in 50% of cases and euthoroidism in the other half.

5. G. The prolonged QT interval in the ECG of patients with Jervell–Lange—Nielsen syndrome results in syncopal attacks or death.

20

1. C. or A. The greater superficial petrosal nerve passes through the Vidian canal to give parasympathetic fibres to the glands of the nose and eye.

2. F. The descendens hypoglossi is joined by the descendens cervicalis to form the ansa cervicalis.

3. G. The lesser petrosal nerve (continuation of Jacobsen's nerve) is a branch of the glossopharyngeal nerve and transmits parasympathetic fibres to the parotid gland.

4. G.

5. G.

21

   1. C.

   2. A.

   3. E.

   4. B.

22

   1. B.

   2. I.

   3. A.

   4. J.

Levels of evidence for studies evaluating therapy, prevention, aetiology or harm:

1a   Systematic review (with homogeneity) of RCTs
1b   Individual RCT (with narrow confidence interval)
1c   All or none†
2a   Systematic review (with homogeneity) of cohort studies
2b   Individual cohort study (including low quality RCT; eg, < 80% follow-up)
2c   'Outcomes' research
3a   Systematic review (with homogeneity) of case-control studies
3b   Individual case-control study
4   Case-series (and poor-quality cohort and case-control studies)
5   Expert opinion without explicit criticav appraisal, or based on physiology, bench research, or 'first principles'
   See <http://www.eboncall.org/content/levels.html>

23

1. A.

2. B.   Although this adult with Down's syndrome may eventually require a BAHA, his most appropriate **initial** hearing aid would be a bone-conduction hearing aid.

3. F.   An elderly arthritic lady is unlikely to be able to manipulate the controls of a conventional BTE aid.

4. D.   For a mild low-tone loss in a young professional, an ITE or in-the-canal (ITC) aid might be appropriate.

24

1. E.

2. F.

3. C.

4. A.

5. B.

Drug volume calculations:
$0.1\% = 1$ mg/ml $= 1:1000$
$1\% = 10$ mg/ml $= 1:100$
$10\% = 100$ mg/ml $= 1:10$

Maximum drug doses:
Lignocaine
Max dose
- Plain $= 300$ mg
- With adrenaline $= 500$ mg

Bupivacaine
Max dose
- Plain $= 175$ mg
- With adrenaline $= 225$ mg

Cocaine
Max dose: 200 mg

Calculations for above question:

1 0.5% bupivacaine with adrenaline.
Max dose = 225 mg
[bearing in mind that 0.5% bupivacaine = 5 mg/ml]
Max dose = 225/5 = **45 ml**

2 0.25% bupivacaine with adrenaline.
Max dose = 175 mg
[bearing in mind that 0.25% bupivacaine = 2.5 mg/ml]
Max dose = 175/2.5 = **90 ml**

3 Dental Xylocaine® = 2% lignocaine + 1:80,000 adrenaline
Max dose = 500mg
[bearing in mind that 2% lignocaine = 20 mg/ml]
Max dose = 500/20 = **25 ml**

4 25% cocaine paste
Max dose = 200 mg
[bearing in mind that 25% cocaine = 250 mg/ml]
Max dose = 200/250 ≈ **1 ml**

5 10% cocaine solution
Max dose = 300mg
[bearing in mind that 10% cocaine solution = 100 mg/ml]
Max dose = 300/100 = **3 ml**

25

1. E.

2. D.

3. B.

4. A.

5. F.

Otomize: Dexamethasone, neomycin, acetic acid
Sofradex: Dexamethasone, framycetin, gramicidin
Gentisone HC: Hydrocortisone, gentamicin
Tri-adcortyl: Triamcinolone, gramicidin, neomycin, nystatin
Otosporin: Hydrocortisone, neomycin, polymixin B
Canesten: Clotrimazole

26

1. and 4. D. Adenoid cystic carcinoma is the most common malignancy of the submandibular, sublingual and minor salivary glands. It exhibits perineural spread, and is associated with slow-growing distant metastases, particularly to the lungs.

2. B. This is a classical history for a carcinoma arising in a pre-existing pleomorphic adenoma.

3. F. SCC is the most likely diagnosis here.

27

1. E.

2. C.

3. B.

4. C.

Choice of statistical test for independent observations

			Outcome variable			
Input variable	Nominal	Categorical (> 2 categories)	Ordinal	Quantitative discrete	Quantitative non-normal	Quantitative normal
Nominal (eg treatment vs placebo)	χ^2 or Fisher's	χ^2	χ^2 trend or Mann–Whitney	Mann–Whitney	Mann–Whitney or log-rank (a)	Student's t test
Categorical (> 2 categories)	χ^2	χ^2	Kruskal–Wallis (b)	Kruskal–Wallis (b)	Kruskal–Wallis (b)	Analysis of variance (c)
Ordinal (ordered categories)	χ^2-trend or Mann-Whitney	(e)	Spearman rank correlation	Spearman rank correlation	Spearman rank correlation	Spearman rank correlation or linear regression (d)
Quantitative discrete	Logistic regression	(e)	(e)	Spearman rank correlation	Spearman rank correlation	Spearman rank correlation or linear regression (d)
Quantitative non-normal	Logistic regression	(e)	(e)	(e)	Plot data and Pearson or Spearman rank correlation	Plot data and Pearson or Spearman rank correlation and linear regression
Quantitative normal	Logistic regression	(e)	(e)	(e)	Linear regression (d)	Pearson and linear regression

(a) If data are censored.

(b) The Kruskal–Wallis test is used for comparing ordinal or non-Normal variables for more than two groups, and is a generalization of the Mann–Whitney U test. The technique is beyond the scope of this book, but is described in more advanced books and is available in common software (Epi-Info, Minitab, SPSS).

(c) Analysis of variance is a general technique, and one version (one way analysis of variance) is used to compare normally distributed variables for more than two groups, and is the parametric equivalent of the Kruskal–Wallis test.

(d) If the outcome variable is the dependent variable, then provided the residuals are plausibly Normal, then the distribution of the independent variable is not important.

(a) If data are censored.

(e) There are a number of more advanced techniques, such as Poisson regression, for dealing with these situations. However, they require certain assumptions and it is often easier to either dichotomise the outcome variable or treat it as continuous.

See: <www.wadsworth.com/psychology_d/templates/student_resources/ workshops/stat_workshp/chose_stat/chose_stat_25.html>.

28

1. E.

2. B.

3. A.

4. G.

The standard error of the mean of one sample is an estimate of the standard deviation that would be obtained from the means of a large number of samples drawn from that population.

A standard deviation is a sample estimate of the population parameter; that is, it is an estimate of the variability of the observations.

A standard error, on the other hand, is a measure of precision of an estimate of a population parameter.

29

1. A.

2. C.

3. B.

4. A.

5. A. or E.

30

1. D.

2. H.

3. A.

4. D.

5. B.

31

1. D. Chagas disease is a parasitic disease caused by *Trypanosoma cruzi*, transmitted by blood-sucking insect vectors (reduviid bugs). Parasympathetic intramural denervation lesions can be dispersed irregularly, leading to dilated oesophagus (mega-oesophagus) or dilated and elongated (dolichomegaoesophagus).

2. C. Patients with achalasia lack noradrenergic, noncholinergic inhibitory ganglion cells, leading to a hypertensive non-relaxed lower oesophageal sphincter.

3. E.

4. B. Scleroderma may be seen as part of the CREST syndrome: Calcinosis; Raynaud's; Esophageal dysmotility; Sceroderma; Telangiectasia.

32

1. F. Pseudostratified non-keratinized stratified squamous epithelium

2. F. Pseudostratified non-keratinized stratified squamous epithelium

3. D. Pavement epithelium without cilia

4. C. Keratinized squamous epithelium

5. E. Pseudostratified ciliated columnar epithelium with goblet cells

33

1. D. This scenario suggests a coagulopathy or thrombocytopenia. Factor assays may be required if the clotting screen is abnormal.

2. H. In this situation, no specific tests of clotting are required.

3. B. The activated partial thromboplastin time (APTT) is used to monitor heparin therapy. If excessively prolonged, epistaxis may occur.

4. G. Alcoholic patients are more likely to have derangement of liver function, causing reduction in clotting factors and low platelet count.

34

1. E. Both erythroplakia and leukoplakia are pre-malignant, but the former is much more likely to undergo malignant change

2. G. Stevens–Johnson syndrome, which is the severe form of erythema multiforme, may be triggered by drugs (especially Septrin), viral infection or food sensitivity. It is associated with characteristic 'target' lesions on the skin, most often on the hands.

3. H. Behçet's disease is a disease of unknown aetiology causing ulcers on the mucus membranes and skin.

4. A. Pemphigoid is due to IgG autoantibodies against basement membrane; it more often affects the elderly.
   Pemhigus is due to IgG autoantibodies against desmosomal components; it more often affects the young, and commonly affects the oral mucosa.

5. G.

35

1. A. Cephalic trimming of the lower lateral cartilages will, with healing, cause the tip to rotate upwards.

2. D.

3. A. The lower lateral cartilages are very superficial and are easily damaged in the initial incisions in an open-approach rhinoplasty.

36

1. C. No investigation is required and if the clinical history is strong enough, the child may be placed on the waiting list for adenotonsillectomy.

2. A. A polysomnogram is useful when central apnoea is suspected: in this case, there will be no respiratory effort when the saturations fall, and this will be detected by the movement sensors on the chest wall.

3. B. Overnight saturation monitoring may be useful if there is any doubt as to whether the child genuinely has OSA.

37

1. B.

2. F.

3. C. The pulsed dye laser has been used in the treatment of skin lesions and more recently in certain conditions of the vocal cords

38

1. B.

2. A.

3. E.

C represents the main lumen of the bronchoscope, and D is the port for introduction of the instruments.

39

    1. D.   Olivary complex

    2. E.   Lateral lemniscus

    3. H.   Inferior colliculus

    4. B.   Cochlear nerve

The mnemonic to remember ABR waves is:
I	**E: E**ighth nerve action potential
II	**C: C**ochlear nucleus
III	**O: O**livary complex
IV	**L: L**ateral lemniscus
V	**I: I**nferior colliculus
VI	Medial geniculate
VII	Auditory radiation (Brodmann's area 41)